510⁶ $25
616.87
Montgomery

Curled corners 10-19 MC

S0-BQZ-275

DISCARD

REEDSBURG PUBLIC LIBRARY
370 Vine Street
Reedsburg, WI 53959

END YOUR
CARPAL TUNNEL PAIN
WITHOUT SURGERY

END YOUR CARPAL TUNNEL PAIN WITHOUT SURGERY

The Montgomery Method

A Daily 15-Minute Program to Prevent and Treat Repetitive Strain Injuries Of the Upper Body - Arm, Wrist & Hand

REEDSBURG PUBLIC LIBRARY
370 Vine Street
Reedsburg, WI 53959

KATE' MONTGOMERY, ND

Sports Touch Publishing

Sports Touch Publishing

Copyright © 2004 by Kate' Montgomery, ND

All rights reserved.
Written permission must be secured from the publisher or author to use or reproduce any part of this book, except for brief quotations in critical reviews or articles.

Sports Touch

Web: http://www.sportstouch.com
Email: orders@sportstouch.com

Published in USA

Library of Congress-in-Publication Data

Montgomery, Kate'

End your carpal tunnel pain -without surgery: a daily 15 minute program to prevent and treat repetitive strain injuries of the upper body - arm, wrist and hand / Kate' Montgomery, ND.

Format and Layout by Stephen Thompson

Text Design by Bruce Gore

Illustrations by Krister Killinger and Oliver Norden

Original Photography by Kate' Montgomery

ISBN-13: 978-1-878069-07-8
ISBN-10: 1-878069-07-8

1. Carpal tunnel syndrome - exercise therapy-handbooks, manuals, etc. 2. Carpal tunnel syndrome-Prevention-Handbooks, manuals, etc. 3. Hand-wound and injuries-Prevention.
2. Title.

Printed in the United States of America
3 4 5 6 7 8 -04 03 02 01 00 3 4 5 6 7 8 –08 07 06 05 04 03 02 01 00

Trauma to the hand and loss of its function is a serious matter. This book is not a medical manual, and the information here is given to help you make informed decisions about health. It is not intended as a substitute for medical treatment. If, after trying these simple techniques, no relief is evident, seek out a chiropractor, osteopath or a physician specializing in the hand.

—————————————

Contents

CONTENTS

- Headaches and Eye Pain, Swelling, Blurry Vision
- Relaxing Your Muscles

CHAPTER 6: *(89 – 110)*
Stretching, Strengthening, and Range-of-Motion Exercises

- Routines to Maintain Proper Alignment
- Why You Want to Warm Up
- Hints for Stretches and Exercises
- Stretching Exercises for the Neck
- Range-of-Motion Exercises for the Shoulder
- Hand-Strengthening Exercises
- Wrists, Biceps, and Triceps Exercises
- Arm-and-Shoulder Strengthening Exercises

CHAPTER 7: *(111 – 124)*
Ergonomics: How to Work Pain-Free

- Setting Up the Work Station
- Work Station Design
- The Importance of Good Posture
- Why You Must Take Breaks
- How to Protect Your Eyes
- Relaxation Techniques for Your Eyes

CHAPTER 8 *(125 – 144)*
A Daily Maintenance Plan: The Twelve-Step Montgomery Method

- Seven Tests for Self-Assessment
- The Montgomery Method
- Forearm Stretch and Release Technique
- Finger Stretch and Strengthening Technique
- Stretching Program
- Muscle-Strengthening Exercises
- Hand Warm-Up and Stretches
- When You Arrive at Work
- Tips For Prevention For The - Computer Programmer, Musician, Golfer, Tennis Player, and Knitter and Needlepointer
- Nutrition and Repetitive Strain Injury (RSI)

CONTENTS

Foreword

With the current health trend of visiting local gymnasiums and being invaded by commercial television to get some other device to improve your abs, it's extraordinary that the one part of your body that you rely on to work and communicate with is taken so much for granted until something goes wrong! Regardless in what capacity you use your hands, whether it be punching stuff into a laptop or being a concert pianist, you'd do well to put Kate' Montgomery's program at the top of your health regimen.

Thanks, Kate' for steering me the right way.

---KEITH EMERSON
keyboardist, Emerson, Lake and Palmer

Acknowledgments

No book is ever the sole essence of one person. My journey to write it was inspired by each person's courage to keep searching. I would like to thank all who have made this book what it is today

I would like to thank all who have made this book what it is today... My daughter who posed for the first copy of this book, never wavered in her support of my beliefs and dreams. My friends Kathy, and Bill, who have always been there for me. My colleagues, Bill, Rick, Esther, Matt, all my teachers and mentors, who taught me a better way to heal... who supported my ideas, and helped me put them into a sound format for the public to understand. John Finch who gave me an incredible gift of the knowledge of herbs in the herbal sports balm. Dr. Jeffrey Anshel for his generous contribution on vision safety, yet another important part to the health of the body. Jim Schmidt, whose research showed that my methods worked and his contribution to this book is so appreciated. Eric Durak, who never lost contact with me, encouraged me to keep going, and to Stephen Thompson, who without his belief in my dreams, passion and that what I had to say had a place in health care, I may never have come back.

I especially want to thank all the people who have so generously written testimonials, because they found this material useful, got better, and were able to return to a functional life again without pain. My sincere thank you and gratitude for your support and for letting me touch your lives.

God Bless you all. May the Light always Shine Upon You.

Kate'

Introduction

Carpal Tunnel Syndrome Is The #1 Crippler Of Our Workforce!

I've met, spoken to, and worked-on as clients, tens of thousands of people who have repetitive strain injuries. I am happy to say that many who tried my program, found relief and returned to a functioning and productive life.

Ten years have passed since the printing of my first edition *of Carpal Tunnel Syndrome, Prevention and Treatment.* The 4th edition was re-titled, *End Your Carpal Tunnel Pain Without Surgery. CTS -* Carpal tunnel syndrome, or WRMSD's - work-related muscular-skeletal disorders, or RSD's - repetitive strain disorders…all are the same term for an injury caused by a repetitive motion. Carpal Tunnel Syndrome, the most widely known, is the #1 reported medical problem. CTS account's for approximately 50% of all work-related injuries according to the 1997-2000 Bureau of Labor and Statistics.

More than eight million people are affected by carpal tunnel syndrome each year. Surgery for carpal tunnel syndrome is the second most common type of musculoskeletal surgery, (back surgery is #1) with well over 230,000 procedures performed annually. ONLY 23% of all carpal tunnel syndrome patients returned to their previous professions following surgery, according to the Bureau of Labor & Statistics and the National Institute for Occupational Safety & Health (1997-2000 Statistics).

Worker's compensation cases of RSD have skyrocketed, and companies, today, feel the strain of this epidemic. Carpal tunnel syndrome costs companies billions of dollars each year in worker's compensation claims, lost revenue and lost workdays. Women account for 45% of the workers, and they experience nearly 2/3rds of all work-related repetitive strain injuries. Thirty-six percent of all carpal tunnel syndrome patients require unlimited medical treatment, according to the National Bureau of Labor and Statistics and National Institute for Health (1997-2000). Unlimited treatment is defined as a possible repeat of the surgery, physical therapy, and/or pain medication. Carpal Tunnel Syndrome surgery deals ONLY with the symptoms, not the cause. Nothing has changed other than to further increase/create the business of carpal tunnel syndrome for the doctors. Various organizations are protecting their interests through ignorance and loss of revenue. Carpal tunnel syndrome is the only surgery that has a "carte blanche" acceptance without first trying non-invasive treatment programs such as chiropractic or muscle therapy. These programs are more cost effective because an employee will have less down time from work and will be able to return to work sooner. The fail rate for carpal tunnel surgery is over 50%. Many times I meet women who have undergone multiple surgeries, still unable to work and struggling with chronic pain.

Why is carpal tunnel syndrome prevalent among the workforce? I believe there are five reasons for this:

1. A lack of education and knowledge about the disorder
2. A failure to understand the body is part of the solution with ergonomics
3. A failure to use alternative medicine therapies as non-invasive and cost effective treatment programs
4. The failure of allopathic medicine, mostly through ignorance, to utilize alternative therapies as a treatment approach
5. Insurance companies, follow outdated regulations without investigating noninvasive options for the patient that keep alternative therapies out of the loop for payment for carpal tunnel syndrome and other musculoskeletal injuries.

Healing a repetitive strain injury is not just a one-time visit – it is a lifetime of maintenance!

Carpal tunnel syndrome does not require a surgical procedure in most cases. The alternative medicine (natural) therapies listed in this book, when applied early, are preventative. An individual, in less time, can be returned to a functional and productive life faster and more reliably, than through an allopathic approach. Because many insurance companies do not compensate for alternative therapies, eight out of ten people using these therapies, pay out-of-pocket to maintain their health and well-being.

The Information Age, a New Century of Promise, Technology - bigger, faster - race, race, race - go, go, go...where does it all end? As we become more and more stationary, the demands on our bodies increase. Work today requires less physical activity, due to technology. Our bodies are moving farther and farther out of balance as we increase stress of less activity with more mental activity, and muscular tension. It never stops! Our job depends on our performance and productivity. The risk is not a risk anymore, it is a reality that someone your know will develop a repetitive strain disorder.

Future Generations…

Children are taught to use a computer as early as two years old. The terms from the '90's, "Nintendo Thumb, Space Invaders Wrist, Gameboy Wrist, Trackball Thumb," are as prevalent today. Computer video games, joy sticks, track balls, keypads, all demand a child to move fast, and to reach awkwardly, to look up, not straight ahead, and to sit on the edge of a chair that does not support or fit their body. Computer classrooms are the norm now. Computer classes are part of their educational curriculum. Children are taught how to use a computer but not to take care of their body or to set up a safe computer workstation. There is little ergonomic support in our schools to protect our child's body when not on the court or playground. The potential for repetitive strain injury during the developmental years is real. Further education on body mechanics and workstation safety is necessary so our children will not suffer the pain of repetitive strain disorder. As I write this, Childhood RSD's are realities. The possibilities of the fullness of life require good health, and technology may rob our children of their future, both in and out of the workplace.

Knowledge of prevention and maintenance techniques, combined with the understanding of what a safe workstation entails, can decrease the risk of repetitive strain injury. The combination of these two effective programs can help stop the carpal tunnel syndrome epidemic from spreading to future generations.

I sincerely hope that the information contained in this book will inspire you to begin a preventive program with continual maintenance for you and your children, before the pain of carpal tunnel syndrome and other repetitive strain disorders robs you and your family of a functional and productive life.

I wish you good luck in your search for the truth. We all deserve the right to a pain free, healthy body and a life full of possibilities!

Kate'

Chapter 1

What is Carpal Tunnel Syndrome

People who have carpal tunnel syndrome can tell you clearly what it is. They can describe the pain and numbness, the difficulty they face in day-to-day life, and the fear that they will no longer be able to do their jobs or the activities they love.

Carpal tunnel syndrome can leave a secretary in tears with pain at the end of the day. It can make a professional guitarist dread picking up his instrument. It can leave a massage therapist ... or a transcriptionist ... or a computer teacher unable to work at all.

However, this condition is treatable and preventable!

WHAT CAUSES CARPAL TUNNEL PROBLEMS

Every day people work at jobs that require them to sit for long hours, push file drawers, bend, lift, and stoop. After a number of years, these positions and movements take their toll on the body. The worker is using his or her muscles, just as an athlete does, but in very specific and sometimes unnatural movements related to the job. Complaints most often heard by employers concern pain in the low back, hip and leg, shoulder, elbow, hand, and wrist. The stress these movements create on the body's muscles and tendons can cause tightness and soreness, which in turn can result in painful trigger points. Trigger points can eventually lead to more serious symptoms such as loss of function and decreased mobility.

Carpal tunnel trauma to the hand can be caused by many factors. Are you a waiter who routinely carries heavy trays on your hand? Do you scrub floors while leaning on the opposite hand? Are you a grocery clerk who repeatedly waves products, one after the other, over an electronic eye? Are you a computer programmer? Baker, golfer, tennis player, carpenter, mechanic, weight lifter, musician, massage therapist, hair stylist, or student? All these careers, and more, can lead to carpal tunnel syndrome.

Carpal tunnel syndrome is common to any profession that involves pinching or gripping with a bent wrist. Blacksmiths used to get this problem long before we had a name for the condition. Pregnant women may also have problems-perhaps because of retaining water and gaining weight but generally the problem disappears after the child is born. People with diseases such as diabetes, hypothyroidism, or rheumatoid arthritis also may suffer from carpal tunnel syndrome. (These conditions, of course, require the care of a physician.)

Studies have shown that a combination of factors such as repetition, force, vibration, and posture increases the risk for carpal tunnel syndrome. Short of stopping the activity that aggravates the condition, carpal tunnel syndrome can be prevented or improved by alleviating muscular tension through implementing a body maintenance program and redesigning tools, work stations, and working methods.

Prevention is the key to strong and stable joints. A body maintenance program

How It All Begun

Many people seem to think that carpal tunnel syndrome and other repetitive strain disorders are conditions of the nineties coinciding, perhaps, with the explosion of personal computers or devices such as grocery store scanners. These conditions have been around for a long time, however.

1850s: In his writings, the physician Sir James Paget discussed median nerve compression in the wrist.

1920s: Meatpackers' hands would swell up like prize fighters', a condition called butchers' wrist. Doctors, in a report on an autopsy, discussed finding damage in the median nerve near the carpal ligament.

1930s: Repetitive strain disorders popped up in farm workers doing repetitive manual tasks.

1950s: Marine sergeants became aware of the condition and mentioned repetitive strain disorders in their journals. George Phalen, M.D., presented a report about compression of the median nerve at the wrist at the annual meeting of the American Medical Association.

1970s: Video games became popular, and children began to develop problems known as Space Invaders' wrist and Nintendo thumb.

1980s: In this decade, there were more and more machines to do work for us, but the result is that we became more stationary, which caused increased stress and tension. Individuals react differently to different work circumstances, however; one person might suffer symptoms after doing a certain job two years, while another might have problems after six months. Because of this, repetitive strain injuries were sometimes not taken seriously.

1990s: As more and more people use personal computers and their mouse pointing devices, more and more have developed carpal tunnel and other problems in the wrist and hand (a problem called "mouse disease" in Norway).

of chiropractic and muscle therapy, along with a daily stretching and strengthening program, prevents the recurrence of carpal tunnel syndrome or any other muscular skeletal injury.

There is NO CURE for carpal tunnel syndrome or any other repetitive musculoskeletal injury, ONLY prevention and body maintenance.

WHO GETS IT

In today's world, many careers-from the most technically advanced to the most routine-create stress on our elbows and wrists. People in any occupation that involves forceful or repetitive use of their hands are at risk of carpal tunnel syndrome. In 1993 the Bureau of Labor Statistics reported that nearly one-third of allworkplace injuries that resulted in lost work days resulted from overexertion or repetitive motion. Nearly two hundred thousand cases were caused by repetitive motion, such as typing, key entry, repetitive use of tools, and repetitive moving of objects. Most injuries affected the wrists.

The bureau also found that the industries with the highest rates of repetitive motion injuries-eight times the rates of all private industry-were clothing manufacturing and manufacturing plants for bags, chips and snacks, cars, and meat packing. Estimates of the cost for time lost from musculoskeletal disorders range from $13 billion to $20 billion a year. In 1994, 13 percent of injuries that caused missed work days resulted from repetitive motion, whether from typing or key entry, repetitive use of tools, or repetitive placing, grasping, or moving objects. The median number of days of work missed was eighteen.

A study in Rochester, Minnesota, suggests that women are developing carpal tunnel syndrome at a greater rate than men-outnumbering them three to one. Not coincidentally, more than three-fourths of women surveyed believed that proficiency and use of devices such as personal computers have helped them get ahead in the workplace.

Since the writing of my last edition five years ago, Carpal Tunnel Syndrome has become the # 1 problem facing the workforce today, costing companies billions of dollars annually in worker compensation claims.

The latest statistics reported by the Bureau of Labor and Statistics and the National Institute for Occupational Safety and Health-NIOSH, (1997-2000) state that Carpal Tunnel Syndrome is the #1 reported medical problem, accounting for approximately 62% of all work-related injuries.

With the increasing stress to perform faster and with the demands on productivity, carpal tunnel surgeries have risen to become the second most performed surgery, and only twenty-three percent of all carpal tunnel syndrome patients were able to return to their previous professions following surgery.

Currently, women account for approximately forty-five percent of our workforce, and they experience nearly 2/3's of all work-related repetitive strain injuries. Thirty-six percent of women receiving carpal tunnel surgery will require unlimited medical treatment.

The current medical treatment plan still only treats the symptoms of carpal tunnel syndrome, not the cause. Muscular skeletal injuries, unless something is broken, can be healed through the use of noninvasive therapies. The use of maintenance therapies such as Chiropractic, massage therapy and Acupuncture can help a person regain a pain-free state where they can continue to be

NEW STATISTICS FROM 1997 TO 2000

- The following sources are compiled from the Bureau of Labor and Statistics and the National Institute for Occupational Safety and Health (NIOSH).
- Carpal tunnel syndrome results in the highest number of days lost among all work related injuries. Almost half of the carpal tunnel cases result in 31 days or more of work loss.- National Center for Health Statistics.
- A report by NIOSH revealed that more than 50% of all food cashiers, (jobs predominantly held by women), suffered some degree of carpal tunnel syndrome and other forms of repetitive strain injuries as a result of the physical demands of scanning products at high speed.
- The U.S. Department of Labor has concluded that Carpal Tunnel Syndrome is the "chief occupational hazard of the 90's"-disabling workers in epidemic proportions.
- Currently, Carpal Tunnel Syndrome affects over 8-million Americans.
- Carpal Tunnel Syndrome is the #1 reported medical problem, accounting for about 62% of all work-related injuries.
- Presently, 25% of all computer operators have Carpal Tunnel Syndrome, with estimates that by the year 2000, 50% of the entire workforce may be affected.
- Only 23% of all Carpal Tunnel Syndrome patients were able to return to their previous professions following surgery.
- Up to 36% of all Carpal Tunnel Syndrome patients require unlimited medical treatment.
- Women are twice as likely to develop Carpal Tunnel Syndrome as opposed to their male counterparts.
- While women account for about 45% of all workers, they experience nearly 2/3's of all work-related Repetitive Strain Injuries.
- Surgery for Carpal Tunnel Syndrome is the second most common type of surgery, with well over 230,000 procedures performed annually.

productive and functional.

Once the body is structurally sound and free of pain, then a stretching and strengthening program can be implemented.

HOW DO I KNOW IF I HAVE CARPAL TUNNEL SYNDROME

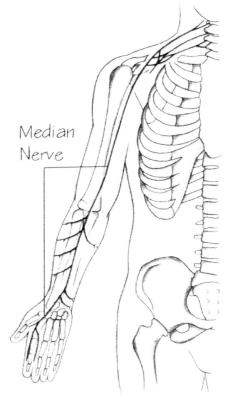

Median Nerve

Carpal tunnel syndrome causes numbness or tingling in your fingers or hand and may cause a pain from the wrist that seems to shoot into your forearm or palm. The pain may be worse at night. *Carpal* is from a Greek word that means "wrist"-and the carpal tunnel is just what it sounds like, a passageway or tunnel through your wrist that protects nerves and tendons. The median nerve, which affects feeling in your thumb and all your fingers except your little finger, passes through the carpal tunnel. When the tunnel becomes swollen, your median nerve is pinched or compressed.

Your Median Nerve

The median nerve, as illustrated on this page, runs from your neck through your shoulder and elbow, ending with the wrist and hand. Entrapment or compression of the nerve can occur at various points. When it occurs in the carpal tunnel of the wrist, it's called carpal tunnel syndrome.

The key to an accurate diagnosis of carpal tunnel syndrome is that the little finger is not affected, because the median nerve isn't connected to this finger. Two simple tests, which are explained in Chapter 2, help diagnose carpal tunnel syndrome. A medical test called an electromyogram will show if electrical impulses going along the median nerve slow down in the carpal tunnel. If they do, your median nerve is probably compressed. This test can be highly invasive and painful, and it can actually prolong the symptoms of carpal tunnel syndrome. An alternative is a device called the Neuronmeter CPT/C that measures nerve sensitivity and may catch problems before they develop into carpal tunnel syndrome. Your health care provider may use this machine to screen for potential carpal tunnel problems. (For more information on Specialty Therapy Equipment, refer to the Resource section of the book.)

Fluctuations in hormone levels that cause swelling or bloating, such as during pregnancy, menopause, or stages of the menstrual cycle, may make carpal tunnel syndrome worse.

Signs and Symptoms

Symptoms of carpal tunnel syndrome may include:

- loss of sense of touch
- tingling and numbness in your hand and fingers
- pain in your shoulder at night, pain in your elbow, or swelling in your wrist area
- loss of grip strength in your hand
- pain in your wrist when you have it stretched in an extreme position (hypertension and hyperflexion), such as holding your hands in a prayer position
- dropping objects more often than usual
- a burning sensation in your wrist and hand area
- being unable to unscrew a jar lid
- finding it difficult to do tasks such as brushing your hair

---

THE PROBLEM WITH CONVENTIONAL TREATMENTS

Standard medical treatments for carpal tunnel syndrome usually begin with rest, and sometimes a doctor may suggest that you wear a wrist splint to keep you from using or stressing the wrist. Often anti-inflammatory drugs such as naproxen, aspirin, *or* ibuprofen, or vitamin B6 are recommended to reduce inflammation. If symptoms continue, a doctor may prescribe an injection of a steroid drug to relieve pain and swelling.

If these treatments don't work, most doctors proceed to surgery. Surgery involves dividing or cutting the transverse carpal ligament that is pressing on the median nerve to relieve the pressure on the nerve. In the 1990s, surgery for carpal tunnel syndrome became the surgery of the decade. This is unfortunate because not only is the operation quite expensive, but it causes loss of the use of the hand for two to six months with no guarantee of post-surgical improvement. (A 1991 study found that surgery did not eliminate all symptoms.)

Surgery is not the answer in 99 percent of cases. The failure rate of surgery is very high. Probably you have known people who have tried surgery for carpal tunnel problems but are still not fully functioning or able to return to their jobs. I'm sorry to say that, in most cases, pain and dysfunction return because of a buildup of scar tissue where the surgery was performed and because the cause of the symptoms was not eliminated. Any relief from surgery-or other treatments-will be temporary as long as the body is misaligned and the person continues to overuse and overstrain the muscles and tendons.

There is always hope, but it all depends on you. It is your responsibility to take charge and become an active participant in healing your body.

NON-CONSERVATIVE TREATMENTS FOR CARPAL TUNNEL SYNDROME & REPETITIVE STRAIN INJURIES

Wrist Splints and Anti-Inflammatory Medication
This approach to treating carpal tunnel syndrome and repetitive strain injuries has a very poor success rate. The FAILURE RATE for total alleviation of all symptoms is about 82.6%.

Lontophoresis and Splints
This procedure is also very ineffective and reveals that only 11 subjects out of 19 experienced relief.

Steroid Injection
The FAILURE RATE for total alleviation after a one-year follow-up is about 75.6% of all patients.

Surgery
The "classic" surgery for carpal tunnel syndrome involves an open technique where a small incision is made over the region of the ligament – which compresses the median nerve. This ligament is released to decompress the median nerve.

The average failure rate, which is very conservative, is 57% after following the patient from 1 - day to 6 - years. At least one of the following symptoms re-occurred during this time; pain, numbness, and tingling sensations. After 6-years, the onset of at least one of these symptoms can reach higher than 90%. Most of these individuals will have surgery more than once, and patients have been known to have as many as five to eight surgeries on just one hand!

7

WHAT THE MONTGOMERY METHOD CAN DO

Many people come to me after reading an article I wrote, wanting to learn why these problems happened to them. Others have had their doctors refer them. Not all of my clients achieved the desired results of full usage, because years of damage had already occurred and they hadn't received the proper treatment. All these people had tried all that traditional Western medicine had to offer. Most had achieved only minimal relief and had not regained even close to full usage of their hands. By the time they left my care, however, they had 80 to 90 percent use of their hands, no matter what their condition had been when they arrived.

Almost all of my clients have returned to their occupation and a pain-free lifestyle. However, they understand it is crucial that they continue to do regular maintenance on their muscles to prevent a recurrence of symptoms.

In most cases, the healing of a musculoskeletal injury is simple. It does take time though and patience on your part, but surgery can be avoided.

Remember, there is no cure for musculoskeletal
injuries – only body maintenance.

I would also like to add this, most people have severe tendinitis not carpal tunnel syndrome. The symptoms may be present – pain, numbness and tingling, but once the structure is realigned and the muscle tension and trigger points are resolved, nerve compression removed, the symptoms disappear.

Any musculoskeletal problem can and will develop into a more severe disorder if action is not taken quickly. Ignoring the pain can only delay healing and recovery. Take care of your body and it will remain pain free and healthy.

HOW ONE WOMAN FOUND RELIEF USING THE MONTGOMERY METHOD

Candace, age forty-seven, the director of a college MBA program for executives, used a computer from four to six hours daily. She also taught classes, which required carrying heavy boxes of materials back and forth, and had many hobbies that she once enjoyed. She had been treated for tendinitis and epicondylitis for three years.

She had seen many physicians, including a general practitioner, a rheumatologist, an osteopath, and a physiatrist (a doctor who specializes in body movement). During those three years, Candace received numerous cortisone shots-which gave temporary relief-and was prescribed several types of anti-inflammatory medicines that eventually caused an ulcer.

Here, in her own words, is her story:

I have experienced severe chronic pain in my arms and elbows for more than three years, which has led to feelings of frustration, depression, and hopelessness. I was searching for a cause and a cure and found it frustrating that not one of my doctors knew either. It took two years for my doctors to acknowledge that my injuries were caused by repetitive strain. By then, of course, the damage was done.

I have taken vitamin B6 supplements, received numerous cortisone shots, and tried every pain-relieving ointment on the market. Two doctors suggested that my only hope for relief would be surgery and a long rehabilitation process. This I wanted to avoid, because

---

Letters from...
A Tapestry Weaver

My hands are essential to the expression of my creativity. Nearly two years ago I had lost most of the use of my right hand. The traditional medical recommendation for the diagnosed carpal tunnel syndrome, surgery, had become my last remaining alternative. In desperation to avoid this solution, I finally went to the library and discovered Kate' Montgomery's book on carpal tunnel syndrome prevention and treatment. Following the recommendations therein I experienced immediate improvement. [By combining] the exercises, Sports Balm, yoga, and massage as suggested, I have [regained] almost complete use of my hand and rarely feel pain. I weave, paint, ski, hike, bake bread, chop vegetables, etc. It is difficult to find words to describe my feelings about my recovery without surgery. Thanks, Kate'

PATRICIA DUNN

everything I had read suggested that I could be worse off after surgery and that there were no guarantees my problems wouldn't be back once I resumed normal activities.

In desperation, fearing that I would soon be unable to efficiently and effectively perform my job duties, I applied for workers' compensation. Thus began my second search for a remedy for my injuries. Although the first doctor again suggested surgery, I told him I wanted to try everything else possible before resorting to such a drastic solution that carried no guarantee for success.

Fortunately, he prescribed physical therapy, and I was thrilled to do something proactive. My fifteen sessions of physical therapy made it possible for me to straighten my left arm-something I could not do when I began treatment-and made me aware of ways to avoid overstraining my muscles. Although I worked hard and religiously attended all the sessions and did my homework assignments, physical therapy alone was not sufficient to provide long-term healing. Attempts to strengthen my muscles as recommended often led to reinjury.

Then I was referred to a truly outstanding physiatrist. By then the pain was beginning to make normal activities almost impossible, and I was having to write all of my documents by hand for my secretary to type-a very inefficient and frustrating setback. I couldn't even do simple household chores. I was depressed and close to giving in to the surgery that I had vehemently avoided for two years.

But on the recommendation of my physiatrist, my workers' compensation gave approval for me to see Kate' Montgomery, a sports therapist specializing in repetitive strain disorder.

When I called to set my appointment, Kate' said, "Don't worry, I can help you." I felt my first glimmer of hope-admittedly darkened by my understandable black cloud of skepticism. After my first session and to my absolute delighted astonishment, I felt better than I had in three years. I have seen Kate' four times and am using the methods she taught me to take responsibility for my own rehabilitation.

Finally, instead of feeling handicapped, unable to do the simple things at work and home I had once taken for granted, I am genuinely on the road to recovery. I am productive in a job that I dearly love. Furthermore, I can now resume the hobbies I had to leave behind three years ago-I even recently refinished furniture! I have my life back and a new way of life now that Kate' has taught me how to take care of myself.

Had I started with Kate's method to begin with, there is no question in my mind that I would have avoided three years of misery, hopelessness, depression, and tremendous expense. I strongly recommend that anyone with repetitive strain injury should not waste a moment's time-they need her help now. We would certainly have a healthier, more productive workforce if our employees were educated in these simple techniques.

HOW CANDACE WAS HELPED

In the beginning I recommended that Candace see a chiropractor specializing in applied kinesiology to make sure her neck and back were aligned correctly.

On her first visit with me she was in a lot of pain, and she was wearing wrist braces to stabilize her wrists. She did have full extension of both arms. Her range of motion-how far she could move each joint-was limited, but not so that it indicated major structural problems. She had numerous painful trigger points, muscle spasms, and knots in her muscles. Her tendons were also inflamed, a condition known as tendinitis.

Before I began muscle therapy, I explained to Candace how her body works and how her bones, muscles, and nerves are interrelated. I explained that when all these are in balance and when there is no tension in the muscles to create a possible misalignment and nerve conductivity problem, the body can then react to its environment without stress or pain.

I began by checking Candace's grip strength using a dynamometer, a device that gauges grip strength. Her grip on both hands was weak for her age.

Muscle testing. I then tested her hand muscles using the thumb and little finger to assess grip strength (a technique called muscle monitoring). I asked her to hold the pads of the thumb and little finger together as I tried to pull them apart (Chapter 2). She could not do this exercise.

This indicated to me a loss of nerve integrity and misalignments somewhere up the path of the arm, not only at the wrist joint. Because I already knew she had pain around the elbow joint, this joint was suspect and could possibly be out of alignment. There were no other joints involved from previous injuries, such as whiplash or shoulder problems.

Realignment. I went to work teaching Candace how to realign her elbows and wrists. Fortunately, her posture was already good. She sat up straight with her shoulders back and down; her head did not jut forward as some people's do, a problem that can cause neck strain or nerve impairment. She was also in good health and did not smoke or drink.

Grip strength. Before we started my twelve corrective steps, I had Candace do a test called the perceived grip strength (Chapter 2). To do this, you squeeze your fingers into a fist as tightly as you can. I asked her to assign a number from one to ten to her effort, with ten representing the strongest. She reported a five for both left and right hands. She found it difficult to make a fist, and her muscles in her arms and hands felt tight when she did so. She described this feeling as "a pulling, like a tension wire."

I directed Candace through the rest of the corrective steps (which are described in Chapters 3 and 4). These involve massaging the muscles of the neck, increasing the range of motion in the shoulder joint, and aligning the elbow joint and the wrist and finger joints. As she did the movements as instructed, to her surprise, her bones began to

---

Dealing with Your Pain

When you have pain and numbness in your hands and wrists, here's what you need to do:

- Be checked by a competent health care specialist to ensure that you have no fractures, dislocations, or other instabilities
- Begin with the self-assessment (Chapter 2) and write your findings n the self assessment sheet at the end of the book
- Next do the twelve-step method to realign joints (Chapter 3). Record your findings
- Heal muscle tissue with muscle therapy, including neurolymphatic massage to speed muscle healing (Chapter 4)
- Use pain relief techniques such as acupressure to speed your healing (Chapter 5)
- Follow a stretching routine (Chapter 6)
- Once healed, do a regular strengthening routine (Chapter 6)
- Warm up regularly (Chapter 6)
- Work at an ergonomically correct work station (Chapter 7).

move. Her elbow bones released and pain began to leave. She then squeezed her wrist together and opened up the joints of her fingers. I tested her grip strength again. Now she was strong-she couldn't believe it had happened so fast. She then did the same steps on the other arm, with the same results. After she did the corrective steps, her perceived grip strength changed, increasing to a level of seven and eight. Her sensitivity returned and she felt a rush of blood to her hand – "like energy moving," she said.

Neurolymphatic massage. Next, I instructed her in neurolymphatic massage (which is explained in Chapter 4). Our lymphatic system is responsible for eliminating metabolic waste products from our body, as well as fighting disease. It is like a garbage or recycling system, taking all the poisons and waste products in the body and filtering them out through the blood system. Every muscle and organ has an associated reflex point. By rubbing these reflex points firmly and deeply, you can effectively flush the lymph fluid from that specific muscle and organ. This strengthens the immune system, decreases pain, and regains muscle strength. It can be done any time and any place.

Muscle therapy. After this we moved on to healing the muscle tissue using muscle therapy, which includes massage. As a muscle therapist, my job is to get the muscles back to normal function. Muscle fibers that have been injured and torn have decreased circulation. Blood flow is diminished, so the muscles aren't getting all the nutrients and oxygen they need to stay healthy. Muscle therapy can change that. With careful and slow working of the muscle tissue, trigger points and muscle spasms will disappear-and your pain along with them.

When you are in a lot of pain, you cannot start hammering deeply into your muscles. It is best to have a professional help you in the beginning. I start slowly doing very specific strokes, spending fifteen minutes on each arm. Then I work the chest muscles and the back and neck muscles to make sure every muscle group that is attached to the arms is pain-free. This takes me approximately one to one and a half hours the first visit.

Stretching. Next came stretching exercises, which were easier for her to do now that her joints were aligned and the muscles less tight. After two weeks, she was able to begin to do strengthening exercises.

Candace was a different person when I finished working with her, and she learned a lot about her body as well. She continues to do muscle therapy and the twelve-step corrective technique because this program is a preventive one. A lack of pain doesn't mean you should stop doing this program.

Candace's story is not unique, it is similar to many I have encountered. The self-care and reeducation program I used with Candace is the same I use with every person I work with and is outlined in this book. Everybody, whether male or female, large or small, weak or strong, is the same in that they all have a skeleton, a nervous system, ligaments, tendons, and muscles. Once you understand the mechanics of your body and the right way to start the healing process, your body, given a chance, will revert to normal function. The age factor comes into play only if you are considerably older and have arthritic problems that contribute to the disorder. Even in these cases, however, using my program can make a difference in the quality of movement and range of motion, and it helps with pain relief.

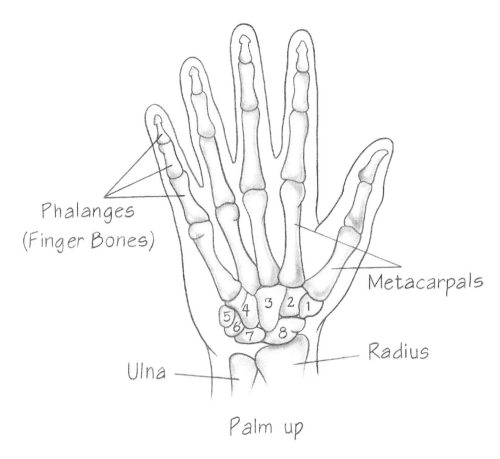

Phalanges
(Finger Bones)

Metacarpals

Radius

Ulna

Palm up

Carpal Bones: (1) Trapezium, (2) Trapezoid, (3) Capitate, (4) Hamate,
(5) Pisiform, (6) Triquetrum, (7) Lunate, (8) Scaphoid

A CLOSE-UP LOOK AT YOUR ARM AND HAND

To understand what can go wrong, it is helpful to understand the structure of your hands and the carpal tunnel itself.

Your hand has eight carpal bones, five metacarpal bones, and fourteen phalanges (the bones of the fingers and thumb).

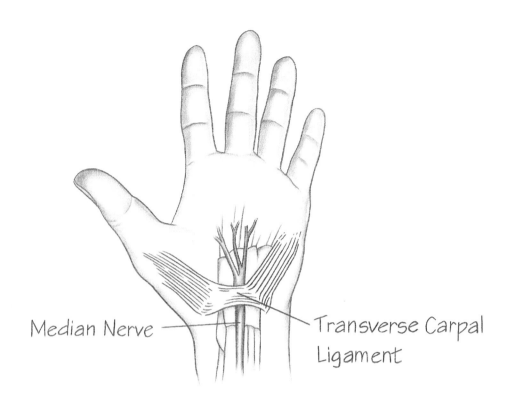

Median Nerve

Transverse Carpal
Ligament

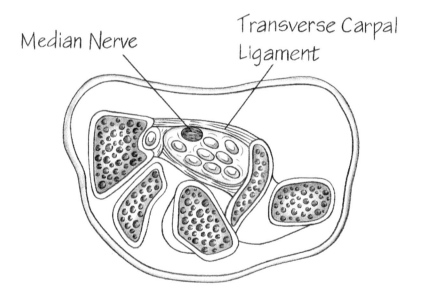

Median Nerve

Transverse Carpal
Ligament

Four bones form the carpal tunnel (these are called trapezium, hamate, pisiform, and scaphoid). The carpal ligament runs between the four bones that make up the carpal tunnel (see illustrations above). The median nerve runs through this tunnel, as do the tendons that flex the fingers.

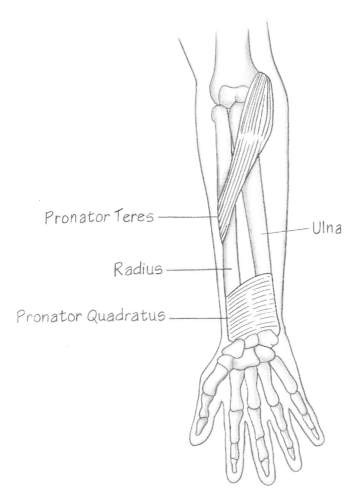

Pronator Teres

Ulna

Radius

Pronator Quadratus

When your arm bones – the radius and ulna – become splayed apart because of a misalignment of your elbow joint, a weakness develops in the pronator quadratus, one of your wrist muscles. As your radius and ulna move apart, the carpal ligament becomes stretched, which puts pressure on the median nerve and the finger flexor tendons of your forearm and hand. This causes pain, muscle weakness, and narrowing of the tunnel pathway. During normal motion, the median nerve moves easily in and out of the carpal tunnel with wrist movement. When the tunnel narrows, it compresses the nerve. The more you flex and extend your wrist, the more the nerve is compressed, eliciting a pain reaction.

THE ORIGINS OF TRIGGER POINTS AND TENNIS ELBOW

One joint that we cannot protect, the one most often ignored, is the elbow. Most of us don't do any exercises to strengthen our arm tendons and muscles. The elbow joint is in constant motion, like a hinge, swinging free. It is the "breaker" between the arm and forearm and has the most stress applied to it. An example of strain to the elbow joint is sitting at a computer, eight hours a day, five days a week, with your elbow bent at a ninety degree angle. Even if your posture is correct, your workstation designed so it is ergonomically correct, and your wrists kept in a neutral position, your elbow joint is compromised by this position. The constant day-to-day movements of the arm, hand, and finger muscles stresses the elbow joint when it is held in one position for a number of hours or when there is direct weight on the elbow and wrist joint.

The constant repetition of a specific motion will cause the muscles of the forearm to become tight, sore, and fatigued from overuse. The strain sets in and painful points called trigger points surface. Trigger points are very sensitive areas that are tender to the touch, and in times of physical or emotional stress, a trigger point may "activate," causing a cycle of spasm and pain. When this happens, the tightness of the tendons and muscles stresses the bones, pulling them out of alignment. When this occurs, nerve entrapment is possible and a pain reaction is elicited.

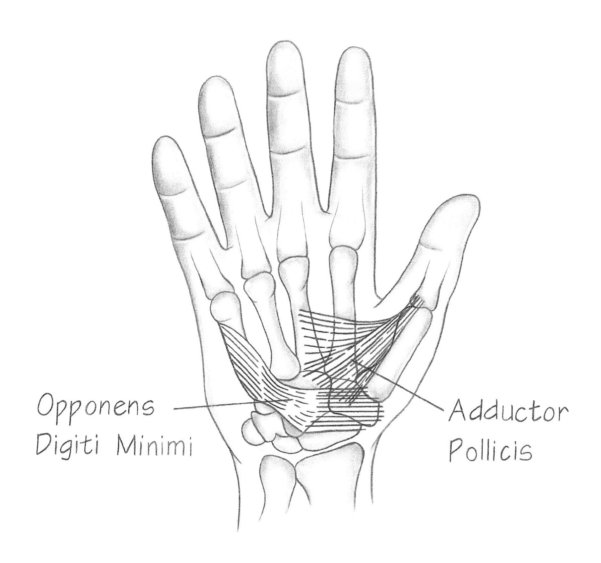

Opponens
Digiti Minimi

Adductor
Pollicis

The adductor pollicis muscle starts at the second and third metacarpal bones and inserts at the base of the thumb. This muscle draws your thumb toward your little finger and helps with the gripping action of your hand. The opponens digiti minimi originates in a fibrous band that covers the carpal tunnel at the wrist. The action of this muscle is to rotate and draw the little finger toward the thumb, and it also helps with the grip of the hand.

The muscles in your forearm that are responsible for the movement that occurs when your arm moves inward (pronation) and when it moves outward (supination) begin at the

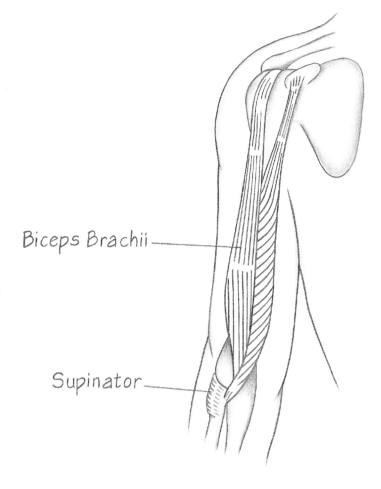

Biceps Brachii

Supinator

elbow joint. When the forearm muscles become overworked and overstrained from constant repetition, the pronator and supinator muscles, flexors, and extensors develop painful trigger points. The muscles, in time, become less flexible, less mobile, and tight and painful to the touch. Misalignment of your elbow joint will increase with the repetitive stress and tension on these muscles. The compromised median nerve, where it passes through the elbow joint, causes pain in the elbow joint, a condition known as pronator syndrome. Tendinitis, a precursor to repetitive strain injuries, can develop, as can epicondylitis (tennis elbow), which involves tiny tears in the tendons and muscles in this area. The procedures explained in Chapters 3, 4, and 5 will help to free up this joint, eliminating pain in the muscles. (See illustrations on previous pages.)

Chapter 2

Do You Have Carpal Tunnel or Another Repetitive Strain Injury?

The number of cases of carpal tunnel syndrome has risen, but the problem is often misdiagnosed. Many people who have symptoms of arm, wrist, and hand pain or numbness have acute to chronic tendinitis with extreme muscle tightness and spasms from overuse and overstrain of the arm. The signs and symptoms of carpal tunnel syndrome vary, and you don't necessarily have pain as an indicator. To date, most people I have screened have had acute to chronic tendinitis – which can lead to carpal tunnel syndrome or other repetitive strain injuries. Only a few have carpal tunnel syndrome or another type of repetitive strain of the upper body.

By using muscle monitoring techniques – also called applied kinesiology – to determine the muscular weakness of your thumb and little finger muscles, you can determine if you have symptoms carpal tunnel syndrome. (Later in this chapter, I will explain how to do these techniques.) Muscle monitoring determines the loss of nerve conductivity and resultant loss of grip strength.

One way to detect a change in the nerve conductivity or electrical flow, other than electromyography, is through muscle monitoring or applied kinesiology. (I believe that electromyograms can cause pain and aggravate and prolong your recovery time.) There is a device called the Neuronmeter CPT/C provides a noninvasive way to determine nerve sensitivity, which can warn of signs of irritation that occur *before* nerve damage. Muscle monitoring, explained later in this Chapter, may show immediate change in the muscular strength of the hand muscles and detect the possible misalignment of the bones involved in the compression or impingement of the median nerve.

People don't understand that not only occupations with repetitive motions can cause repetitive strain injuries such as carpal tunnel syndrome, but normal everyday life can also contribute. It's only since computers have come into common use that repetitive strain injuries have come to our attention.

Once carpal tunnel syndrome or another repetitive strain injury has been determined, you can begin following the program outlined in this book. It will restore vital energy and sensation in your nerves, rebuild strength in your hands, relieve existing problems, and help prevent future problems. In many cases you will find at least some immediate relief.

SEVEN TESTS TO DETERMINE IF YOU HAVE CARPAL TUNNEL SYNDROME OR REPETITIVE STRAIN SYMPTOMS

Here are seven quick and easy techniques you can use to help determine if you have carpal tunnel symptoms. At the end of this book there is a Self-Assessement Sheet, record your results and keep track of your improvement.

TEST 1. TINEL'S TEST

In this test you hold one hand out, palm side up, and tap the carpal ligament over the median nerve as shown. This nerve is at the crease of the wrist, between the middle of the hand and thumb. Pain or a tingling sensation indicates carpal tunnel syndrome or nerve entrapment. Record your findings.

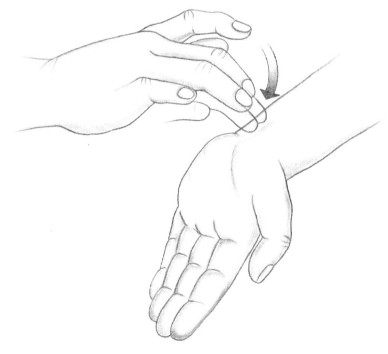

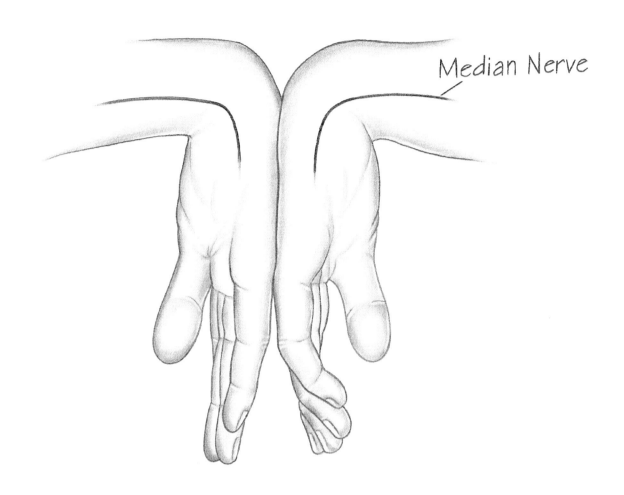

Median Nerve

TEST 2. PHALEN'S TEST

In this test you deliberately hyperextend your wrists. Hold your hands down and press the back of your hands together and hold for a minute. If you begin to feel numbness or tingling, that means you have pressure on the median nerve, which can indicate a possible misalignment problem and a symptom of carpal tunnel syndrome. Record your findings.

TEST 3. MUSCLE MONITORING – DO YOU HAVE A MISALIGNMENT?

The following tests will determine if the bones in your wrist and elbow joint are misaligned, or if you have some misalignment in your neck and shoulder area. Neck and shoulder misalignment may result from previous back, shoulder, or neck injuries, such as whiplash in a car accident, or from positioning your body in an incorrect posture for many years, such as hunching over a keyboard or desk. All these problems can cause a loss of nerve conductivity and muscular strength in your hands.

To do these simple tests, called muscle monitoring, you need a friend to help.

1. Place the pads of your thumb and little finger together, palm side up, and have a friend try to pull the thumb and little finger apart. Your friend should pull lightly from the base of your thumb and the little finger joint.

2. Now place the pads of your thumb and little finger together, palm side down, and have a friend try to pull your thumb and little finger apart. Your friend should pull lightly from the base of your thumb and the little finger joint.

If in both tests your fingers come apart easily, you may have a misalignment. Record your findings.

If your fingers hold strong, however, you should still do the twelve-step method in Chapters 3 and 4, as there is always room for improvement and this program also works to help prevent misalignments and other problems. It's a matter of prevention and body maintenance – and well worth your time.

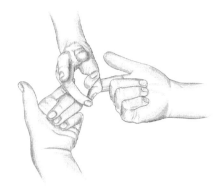

Palm side down

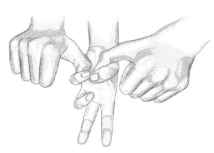

Palm side up

TEST 4. FINGER PAD SENSORY PERCEPTION OF TOUCH

The loss of our sense of touch comes upon us so fast that in most cases we didn't know we had lost it. This test is about discovering your innate sense of touch and using your intuitive perception, you determine what you FEEL is your level of Sense of Touch is.

A person's innate sense of perception or feeling can be traced back to their knowledge of how they feel when healthy or ill. This has been developed over their life span. "I feel sick today, my back hurts, I just don't feel just right." I am sure we have all heard these statements or even said them ourselves.

Our sense of awareness can be heightened if we understand how to interpret it. Sensory perception is our level of awareness based on our frequency of the arriving action potentials. In the case of the touch sense, the amount of pressure brings a conscious awareness of a sensation, which is our perception at that moment. In most cases, when a learned perception is taught and brought to an individual's attention, they become more aware of how to perceive changes in their body.

Sensory Perception...

Sensory receptors represent the interface between the nervous system and the internal and external environments. A sensory receptor is a specialized cell that monitors conditions in the body or the external environment. When stimulated, a receptor passes information to the Central Nervous System (CNS) in the form of action potentials along the axon of a sensory neuron. The arriving information is called a <u>sensation</u>.

The term "general senses" refers to sensations of temperature, pain, pressure, vibration and proprioception (body position). General sensory receptors are distributed throughout the body and they are relatively simple in structure. Some of the information they send to the CNS reaches the primary sensory cortex and over conscious awareness. Sensory information is interpreted on the basis of frequency of arriving action potentials. For example, when pressure sensations are arriving, the harder the pressure the higher the frequency of action potentials. The conscious awareness of a sensation is called a perception. (Martini)

25

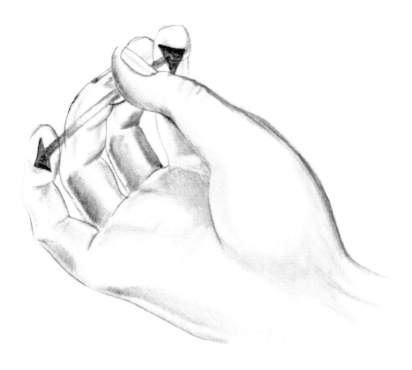

To determine what your level of fingerpad sensitivity is, first close your eyes. Then gently rub the tips of the finger pads with your thumb. Use your perception of touch to determine what level of sensitivity you FEEL you are at. This is your perception, not anyone else's. Don't think too hard on this. Your first impression is the most accurate. Now give yourself a number between 1 and 10, where 10 is the most sensitive, how sensitive to touch do you FEEL? Record your findings.

TEST 5. PERCEIVED GRIP STRENGTH ASSESSMENT

A physician or chiropractor will use a dynamometer, a device with a gauge attached, which you squeeze to test your grip strength. If you don't have access to a dynamometer, however, a simple method of squeezing your fists together can help you determine your current perceived grip strength. You can use this again later to see how your strength has improved.

Squeeze your fists firmly together, one at a time, and give yourself a number from one to ten that you believe measures your grip strength, with ten representing the strongest. Squeeze each hand separately. How strong does each hand feel? What is your perception of your grip strength? (If you are shaking to be strong, it means that there is a "short in the system and you have to try really hard to be strong). Record your findings.

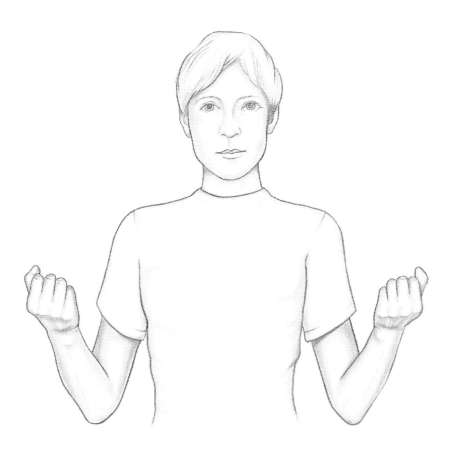

TEST 6. MUSCLE PALPATION FOR TIGHTNESS

PRESS and **PROBE.** Use your fingers to determine if there is muscle and tendon pain. Press into the belly of the forearm muscle and up around the elbow joint where the tendon attaches to the bone. Rub the muscle back and forth, against the grain of the muscle. Can you feel the "ropiness" of the muscles? Is their pain? If there is pain near the joint (elbow), you may have inflammation of the tendon or tendinitis. If there is pain in the belly of the muscle, you could have what are called trigger points. Record your findings.

Trigger Points – X's

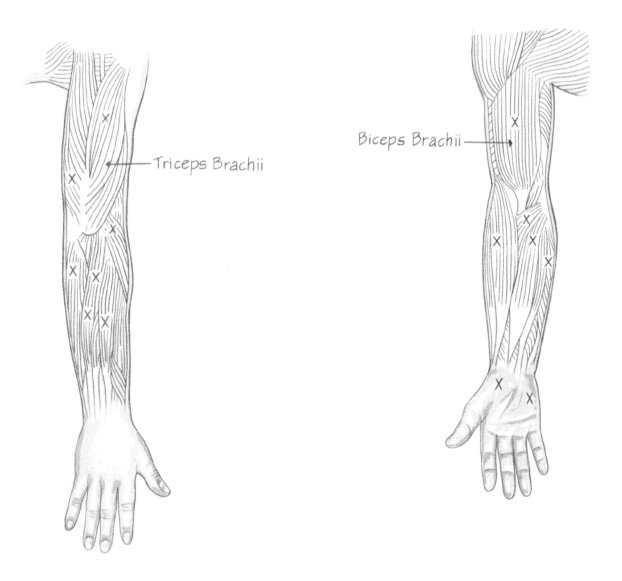

TEST 7. PAIN

Pain is an indicator that something is wrong and out of balance in your body. Ignoring this signal, or taking drugs to cover up this symptom, could lead you down an unknown road that could take you longer to uncover and rid your body of the true cause. Listening to your pain is the best way to begin to uncover a disease process in your body. Rate your pain level: One to ten, ten the most pain, record your pain level. Later after doing the twelve-step program, rate your pain level again. You should see a difference.

Once you have done your self-assessment, and written down your findings in the self-assessment sheet provided at the end of this book, proceed next to The Twelve-Step Montgomery Method. Read how to do each of the corrective exercises described in Chapters 3 and 4. Afterwards, repeat the seven tests to see if you have improved. Record your findings. Remember, this is only the beginning and it may take several sessions to reach a symptom-free body.

If you have shown any improvement, then follow the healthcare protocol I have recommended as a course of treatment and preventive maintenance. Ultizing these practitioners along with your self-care program will help your body return to a healthier state of function and to a productive life faster.

I recently read a booklet by Dr. Walter H. Schmitt, (D.C, D.I.B.A.K., D.A.B.C.N.) titled *Stop Your Pain Now*. It is a great self-help book. It was written for the lay person as well as the practitioner. It is easy to read and follow the instructions. (Refer to the Resource section to find out how to order this booklet.)

HEALTH CARE PROTOCOL: WHO TO SEE WHEN?

When you begin to have pain or numbness, you should first see a physician specializing in the hand. They can rule out possibilities of a broken bone or a tumor, cyst, or nerve ganglion (a knot-like mass of nerve cells) that can cause pain and obstruction of the nerve pathway to the hand. A physician can also diagnose problems such as rheumatoid arthritis or bursitis that may be causing pain.

After the visit with the physician, you may choose to visit other health care professionals for help with pain relief. Use all practitioners with common sense, and don't ignore what your body is telling you. Here's a rundown on techniques you may find useful.

Chiropractic. A chiropractor is trained in the physical manipulation of the spine and joints of the body. Adjusting the alignment of the bony structure improves the flow of nerve impulses to the brain and restores strength to the muscles. My recommendation is to find a chiropractor who specializes in applied and clinical kinesiology. Chiropractic is very effective in releasing the stress and tension of the ligaments, tendons, and muscles from the attaching bones. This will ensure that the alignment will hold longer and maintain nerve integrity to the musculature. After muscle therapy, visiting a chiropractor may be useful. At this point your muscles will be relaxed. If needed, the therapy is easier for a chiropractor to adjust your spine and joints when there is less tension in your muscles. If you maintain your muscles through consistent muscle therapy and self-care, when the initial sessions are over, you may want to visit a chiropractor once a month or every two to three months for maintenance care, depending on what type of work and other activities you do.

Muscle therapy. Massage of your muscles from a well-trained, licensed massage therapist or practitioner versed in muscle therapy can relax the muscles, increase circulation, release tension buildup, speed recovery time, and relieve pain. In the beginning you may need to have your muscle tissue worked on by a professional to relieve tension, painful spasms, and trigger points. Optimally, you would meet with a therapiest once a week for the first month and then twice a month in conjuncton with your self-care program. The amount of muscle therapy needed depends on the soft tissue damage, and maintenance depends on the workload your occupation

---

Letters from...
A Medical Transcriptionist

I am a career medical transcriptionist who has seen many co-workers lose their ability to continue in their careers because of carpal tunnel syndrome and overuse syndrome. The forward arm extension and the lateral arm extension exercises, I couldn't help but notice, gave me immediate and really rather miraculous relief – such simple movements! The miraculousness of the forward arm extension and the lateral arm extension give me confidence in the longer term effects. Thanks again, Kate'

JANE DANIEL

puts on your muscular system. You should be able to relax and breathe easily during a session. If you cannot do this, tell your therapist to lighten up. Remember to tell the therapist how you are feeling. If you have never had this type of therapy before, the first session may be uncomfortable. You are getting used to the therapist, and so is your body. The therapist is having to go through many layers of tension and pain to achieve a better range of motion. The second session will be better. Remember that your muscles are feeling discomfort because they are going through the healing stage to become pain-free.

Acupuncture. An acupuncturist is a trained practioner of oriental medican. Herbal and needle therapy, with needles put into specific points in the skin, is used to help with pain relief and to restore balance and vital energy. Many people find that this makes them feel more relaxed and calmer mentally. Monthly visits are recommeded for stress reduction and mental and physical relaxation.

Physical therapy. A physical therapist can recommend exercises for rehabilitation to strengthen the muscles of your neck, shoulders, back, arms, and hands. Physical therapists can help relieve pain through muscle-strengthening exercises, stretching, applications of hot and cold, ultrasound treatments, or relaxations techniques. They can also guide you in knowing how to help yourself and can design individualized exercises. Remember to ask questions about the therapy recommended for rehabilitation. Usually you need a doctor's referral to see a physical therapist.

Other people you may want to visit are a nutritionist, who can design a program for your particular body type, and an herbalist, for natural remedies and anti-inflammatories.

How to Find Good Care

As with all health care professionals, choose wisely. Get a recommendation from a friend or doctor, and check credentials or references. Spend time interviewing a prospective practitioner; don't be afraid to ask questions. You should feel comfortable with the environment in which the treatment will take place. Mental relaxation is just as important as physical relaxation, as it's difficult to achieve one without the other. You are responsible for taking care of your body and choosing whom you allow to work on it to help you stay healthy.

Acupuncturist. To find a licensed acupuncturist, check with the National Commission for the Certification of Acupuncturists at (202) 232-1401. The American Academy of Medical Acupuncture, at (800) 521-2262, can refer you to a medical doctor with training in traditional acupuncture.

Chiropractor. For problems related to musculoskeletal injuries, you want a chiropractor who specializes in applied and clinical kinesiology. A chiropractor should have six years of training at the college level at a recognized chiropractic school and a state license. Applied and clinical kinesiology are techniques learned outside chiropractor school and are specialized training. To locate a chiropractor who specializes in applied kinesiology, contact:

- The International College of Applied Kinesiology, USA
  6405 Metcalf Avenue, Suite 503 Shawnee Mission, KS 66202
  (913) 384-5336; web site - www.icakusa.com
- International Chiropractic Pediatric Association (icpa)
  http://www.icpa4kids.com; email: info@icpa4kids.com

Massage or muscle therapist. To locate licensed therapists in the United States, you can contact:

- American Massage Therapist Association: Find a therapist - (888) THE-AMTA, (800) 843-2682
  Web site: www.amtamassage.org; Email:infor@amtamassage.org
- Associated Bodyworkers and Massage Professionals: (800) 458-2267, (800)667-8260 Fax; Web
  site:www.abmp.com:; Email: expectmore@abmp.com
- International Massage Association, Inc.: (540) 351-0800; Web site: www.imagroup.com

For Canadian therapists, contact:

- Massage Therapist Association of Alberta: (403) 340-1913, (403) 346-2269 Fax; Email:
  mtaa@telusplanet.net
- Massage Therapist Association of British Columbia: (604) 873-446; Email:
  mta@massagetherapy.bc.ca
- Massage Therapist Association of Manitoba, (204) 254-0406, (204) 668-0951 Fax
- New Brunswick Massotherapy Association, Inc., (506) 459-5788, (506) 459-5788 Fax
- Newfoundland Labrador Massage Therapist Association, (709) 726-4006, (709) 754-0123 Fax
- Massage Therapist Association of Nova Scotia, (902) 429-2190
- Prince Edward Island Massage Therapy Association, (902)368-8140, (902) 368-6524 Fax
- Ontario Massage Therapist Association, (416) 968-6487, (800) 668-2022, (416) 968-6818 Fax
- Federation Quebepoise des Masseurs et Massotherapeutes, (514) 597-0505, (800) 363-9609 Fax
- Saskatchewan Massage Therapist Association, (306) 384-7077, (306) 384-7175 Fax

Physical therapist. A qualified physical therapist has a bachelor's or graduate degree in physical therapy and a physical therapy license. Before choosing a physical therapist you may want to ask if the therapist has treated people with your problems before and what treatment plan is recommended. In some states you can directly visit a physical therapist, at least for an evaluation, but in many you need a doctor's referral before any treatment can begin. Contact the American Physical Therapy Association at www.apta.org.

Physician. You need a physician who specializes in the care of the hand and upper extremities. For a referral, call the American Medical Association in your state.

WHEN IT'S NOT CARPAL TUNNEL

A number of other conditions can cause symptoms that you may mistake for carpal tunnel syndrome or another repetitive strain injury. Here's a rundown on seven of these conditions.

Bursitis. Until something goes wrong, you probably won't know you have a bursa. There are about 150 of these tiny liquid-filled sacs in your body, which serve as little pillows to cushion your muscles and tendons. When they're injured from a blow, a fall, or too much constant pressure, they swell painfully. Kneeling or leaning on your elbow too long can cause bursitis, as can badly fitting or poorly designed shoes. Occasionally, bursitis is caused by an infection or by a nearby swollen tendon. It can cause dull pain that gets worse when you move your joint, and it may wake you up at night.

The conventional treatment for bursitis is rest and ice. Many physicians recommend that you stop the activity that causes pain, apply ice packs for twenty minutes every hour or two, and after forty-eight hours switch to heat, such as a warm bath or a hot compress for pain relief. I recommend gentle massage to the muscles around the joint to increase circulation and to decrease inflammation. Physicians will warn you, however, that directly massaging the inflamed bursae will only make them worse, as pressure is what caused the problem in the first place.

Tendinitis. Tendons are bands of tissue that connect your muscles to your bones. Tendinitis or inflamed tendons is caused by stress on a tendon, such as misalignments or micro-tears. Tendinitis can be felt in the joints of the ankle, shoulder, elbow, wrist, hand, or hip. Because tendons and bursae are so close together, when tendons swell they can put pressure on the bursae, so you may often have both conditions at the same time, particularly in the shoulder. Treatment consists of alignment and muscle therapy. You shouldn't exercise until you're recovered, but you need to run the affected joint gently through its range of motion to retain flexibility. Massage lightly to increase circulation and to decrease swelling.

Epicondylitis. This is also known as tennis elbow or golfer's elbow. The small knobs at the end of your humerus, the main upper arm bone, are known as epicondyles, and overworking the wrist and fingers can stress or tear the muscle and tendon at this spot. Symptoms of epicondylitis can include pain in the forearm and hand numbness, and pain on the inside or outside of the elbow joint (typically worse when you bend your wrist). When your elbow is out of

33

alignment, this problem can surface because of the constant repetitive stress on the elbow joint from using it in a specific motion. Generally, with this condition you will feel pain if you try to straighten your arms, and the elbow area may hurt when you touch it. For this, try the elbow alignment exercises explained in Chapter 3 plus massage.

Raynaud's Disease. Raynaud's has symptoms like those of carpal tunnel syndrome, but it is not a repetitive strain injury. It involves a constriction of the blood vessels and has been linked to arthritis, lupus, and other problems, such as using hand tools that vibrate. Raynaud's causes cold fingers and sometimes tingling and numbness.

Sprain. Ulnar collateral ligament sprain is the most common hand sprain. It is when the ligaments at the base of the thumb (MP) joint are torn or partially torn. This condition occurs when a ligament is stretched beyond its normal limits. This "type" of sprain often happens while playing sports. Most people think of the term "Sprain" as a generic term for any minor injury to the extremities, lessening the impact of its seriousness. Treatment of a sprain should be immediate. (Read the section on Herbal Sports Balm – it works wonders to help heal sprains).

***The most common injuries seen today are with children and teens- where the result is from in-line skating accidents. Do as the experts do, wear protective equipment, i.e. wrist protectors, elbow pads, knee pads, and a helmet. (APTA)

Trigger Finger. This is brought on by continually grasping an object such as in manufacturing. The "repetitive" reaching for an object and grasping it with your hand eventually leads to tendinitis, inflammation of the flexor tendons in any or all of the fingers and thumb. This condition can become serious if not taken care of immediately. The finger may elicit a clicking or popping noise and it can lock in place. To avoid serious damage, seek medical care. (APTA)

DIP Joint. This stands for "distal interphalangeal joint" and are the finger joints closest to the fingernails. It is the tearing of the tendon that can cause the finger to droop. DIP joint injuries are common in sports, occurring most often when a baseball, basketball or volleyball jams into the end of the finger, injuring the DIP joint. To avoid serious damage, seek medical care. (APTA)

OTHER REPETITIVE STRAIN INJURIES

As I've mentioned, carpal tunnel syndrome, while the best known repetitive strain injury, is certainly not the only one. There are other conditions, some with similar symptoms, and you can have more than one at a time.

While the twelve-step method and the other techniques presented in this book will likely give relief for most repetitive strain injuries, you may need professional medical counsel for diagnosis or to determine the seriousness of the muscle strength loss or to see if you have any other injuries.

Here's a look at other repetitive strain problems.

Cervical radiculopathy. This compression is caused by holding a phone with an upraised shoulder. It affects discs in your neck and makes moving your head painful. Symptoms include weakness in the upper arm and shoulder and, possibly, numb fingers. Preventing this is simple: If you need your hands free while you are talking on the phone, use a phone support, phone headset, or speaker phone.

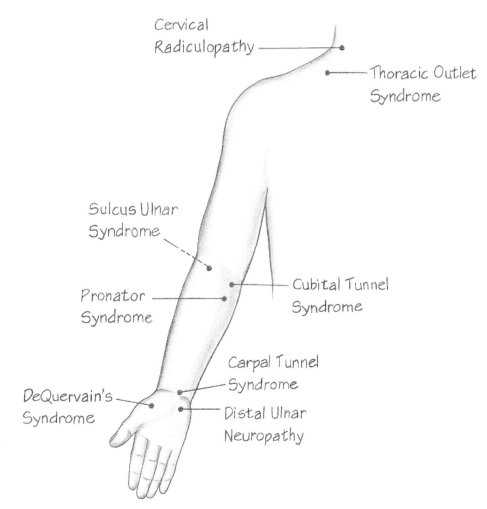

Staying Healthy

Although we all have the same components making up our bodies, each person's body is unique. Healing time from repetitive strain injuries depends on how the individual body responds, and how willing you are to do the exercises in the program outlined for you. It is important to remember that symptoms can return if you overuse your body.

To make this clearer, think of people who run marathons. They train diligently so they can compete in their 26.2-mile event without developing an injury. But what if they ran a marathon every day?

Even the most superbly trained body cannot hold up under those strenuous demands. It would break down and become injured. The same is true of our arms. Marathon sessions of nonstop keyboarding, quilting, or glass blowing will cause injury because of the demand for our arms to perform at a level they cannot achieve and remain healthy.

DeQuervain's Syndrome. When a tendon rubs against the lining of a joint, called the synovia, the resulting inflammation is called tenosynovitis. DeQuervain's, a type of tenosynovitis, is an inflammation of the tendon and the tendon sheath at the base of the thumb. It can be caused by using a track ball on a keyboard, banging too hard with your thumbs while you type, or by jamming the joint accidentally. The result is sharp pain when your thumb is moved or twisted.

Pronator Syndrome. This condition, like carpal tunnel syndrome, involves compression of the median nerve, but in this case it's at the pronator teres muscle – a muscle that twists the forearm and helps the elbow bend. It involves pain in the wrist and forearm, and Phalen's and Tinel's tests are negative. It can happen at work when your elbows are regularly raised too high (such as reaching up to use a computer mouse), or held at an awkward angle.

Ulnar Nerve Problems.

Cubital tunnel syndrome. This affects anyone who works with a bent elbow and makes small movements while holding a tool or device. It may result in numbness, tingling, and eventual weakness in the affected muscles, caused by entrapment of the ulnar nerve in the underarm. People who get this commonly include dentists, musicians, chefs, jewelers, or anyone who writes a lot.

Distal ulnar neuropathy. Also called Guyon's canal syndrome or ulnar tunnel syndrome. What happens here is that the wrist's ulnar nerve, which is in a tunnel near the carpal tunnel, becomes compressed. This can cause numbness in the ring and little fingers, and problems grasping.

Sulcus ulnar syndrome. You may know your ulnar bone as your funny bone, and this condition can develop in people who frequently lean on their elbows. It can cause numbness, tingling, or even a contraction in the ring and little fingers.

Thoracic Outlet Syndrome. These symptoms are caused by compression of the nerves that pass into the arms from the neck. This situation occurs when there is a misalignment of the lower cervical and upper thoracic vertebrae. It can be caused by an extra rib, a broken collarbone, or rounded shoulders from poor posture. Thoracic outlet syndrome causes pain, weakness, numbness, and tingling in the shoulder, arm, hand, or all three. Hand pain is often the worst in the ring finger and little finger, and pain gets worse as you use the arm. Musicians such as guitar players who sit with rounded shoulders, hunched over and looking down for long periods of time, tend to get this condition, as do students who hunch over their books, a knitter, or a person who quilts.

Ganglion Cyst. What it is and how to treat it. Ganglion cysts are the most common masses seen in the hand and wrist. They usually appear on the back of the wrist, but can also occur on the palm side or at the base of the fingers. They are formed from tissue, which lines the joints or tendons, and when irritated, will fill with fluid. They can increase in size during periods of irritation and often resolve spontaneously. Ganglion cysts are not tumors and are not cancerous. They are soft and pliable. When the cyst is small and painless, simple massage over the cyst will help to disperse the fluid. When the joints of the arm (elbow and wrist) are out of alignment, it makes the possibility that fluid can be trapped and a cyst can form. If the cyst continues to enlarge, you should seek out a practitioner such as a Chiropractor to help in the realignment of the joints and then a massage therapist to help with the muscle strain/overuse, which has brought on the cyst.

Ganglions can be painless; however, they often are associated with tenderness and pain and can restrict the range of movement. The cause of ganglions is not always clear. Occupational factors can play an important role in the development of ganglions. Occupations that require workers to excessively overuse certain joints such as the wrist and fingers pose the most risk for the development of a ganglion cyst.

When a ganglion cyst is taken care of early on, it does not require a surgical procedure. Prevention and maintenance is the key factor in avoiding a ganglion cyst.

Double Crush Syndrome. A double crush syndrome is a compression of nerves in two separate areas, usually distant from the other. The nerve is "crushed", "compressed" or irritated in the spine. This is preparing the more distal areas of the nerve for dysfunction when that part is eventually stressed (double crush). Many of the client's who have come to me for carpal tunnel, usually complain of neck, (whiplash) shoulder and upper back pain also. I usually ask them if they have had a car accident, taken a fall, anything that could have affected their upper body. Poor posture and stress are also are factors that affect our body and can compromise the integrity of the spine.

Letters from...

One Woman's Experience with CTS

In October of 2003, 3 months after completing chemotherapy and radiation for breast cancer on my left breast, I developed symptoms of CTS on the right hand and wrist. At the end of Nov, I saw an orthopedic doctor who did nerve conduction studies a week later and referred me to a hand surgeon. While I was waiting for my appointment with the surgeon I happened to learn what was involved with carpal tunnel surgery and for the first time, I heard that it is not always desirable.

I found Kate' Montgomery's book at my local library by chance and started to do the 12 steps described in her book. Within a few days the numbness in my fingers went from constant to intermittent, and by the time I met with the surgeon in January the symptoms were gone. The surgeon evaluated the nerve conduction studies and recommended surgery. I showed her Kate's book and said I would like to continue with the exercises. The doctor agreed if I would come back in a month for a check. I recently had that check-up and my symptoms had not returned. I have been discharged from the surgeon's care with the understanding I will self-monitor my condition.

Judy Kuhn
March, 2004

P.S. During my last appointment, Dr. Brown said she has had three other patients in the intervening month who requested alternatives to surgery.

Chapter 3

The Montgomery Method: Twelve Easy Steps for Prevention and Treatment

We use our bodies continually. Through our brain, our nervous system signals our muscles to move in whatever direction we choose. This is normal. Unfortunately, few of us have been taught how to care for our bodies from a mechanical viewpoint. It is time we learned. My method integrates three systems – the skeletal, muscle and nervous systems. Together, they work in unison to create harmony and balance. When one of the three systems moves out of alignment or becomes compressed or over-strained, it affects the other two. Over time, this can cause pain and tension in our body. My method addresses this balance of the whole body within these three systems.

THE MONTGOMERY METHOD

The Montgomery Method is a twelve-step practical program of self-correction to align your joints and restore energy and strength to the muscles. It also includes exercises and stretches that you can incorporate into your life, anytime and just about anywhere. This program is designed to help you regain mobility and to support and stabilize the muscles and joints of the arm, wrist, and hand.

When you begin to restore balance to the body by increasing blood flow, eliminating the pain and releasing muscle tension, you will feel the reemergence of your sense of touch and strength in your upper body, but particularly in your arms and hands. After doing the restorative movements, the tendons and muscles around your elbow and wrist joint may feel sore the next day. That's because your elbow bones, as well as the tendons and muscles that support and hold the joints together, will be back in the correct alignment. With the aid of muscle therapy, muscle soreness, trigger points, and pain will disappear.

STEP 1: POSTURE CORRECTION

The first step is to correct your posture. This is an ongoing process, especially if you're used to sitting or standing incorrectly as in the illustrations on this and following pages. At first, the correct position may feel unnatural, and you may have to do frequent self-checks in a mirror, if possible to ensure that you are keeping your spine and neck aligned correctly.

Habits acquired at home or at work can cause recurrent minor injuries to the neck joints. Continual irritation can inflame the nerve, causing pain in your neck, shoulders, arms, and hands. Sit tall, with your head erect on your shoulders and your eyes straight ahead. Move your shoulders back and down.

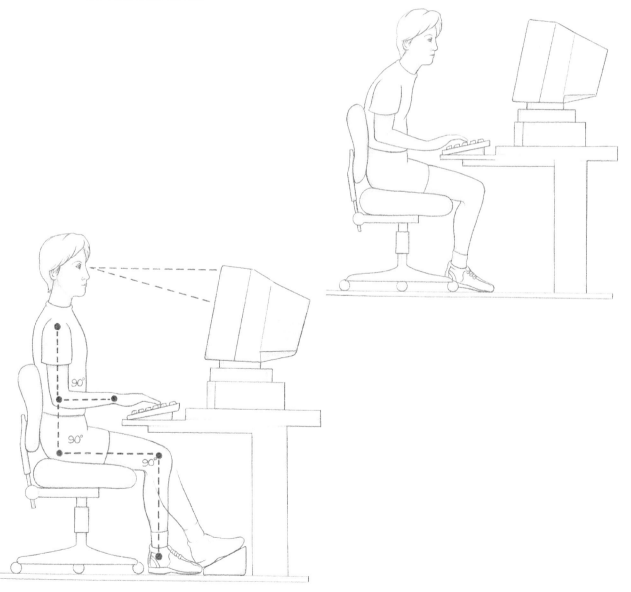

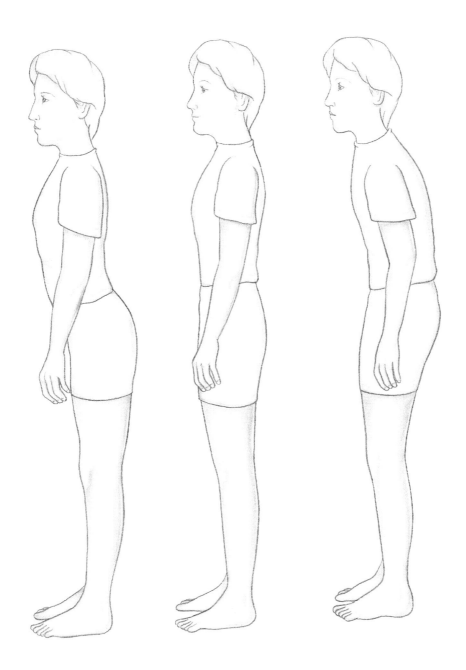

When you are standing, be careful not to over extend your lower back or lock your knees, as in the first illustration above. You should also be aware of your shoulders, preventing them from hunching over, as in the third illustration above. Correct posture is demonstrated in the center illustration. Your back should have a natural curve and your pelvis should be tucked slightly under. Raise your height from your rib cage, drop your shoulders and relax your knees.

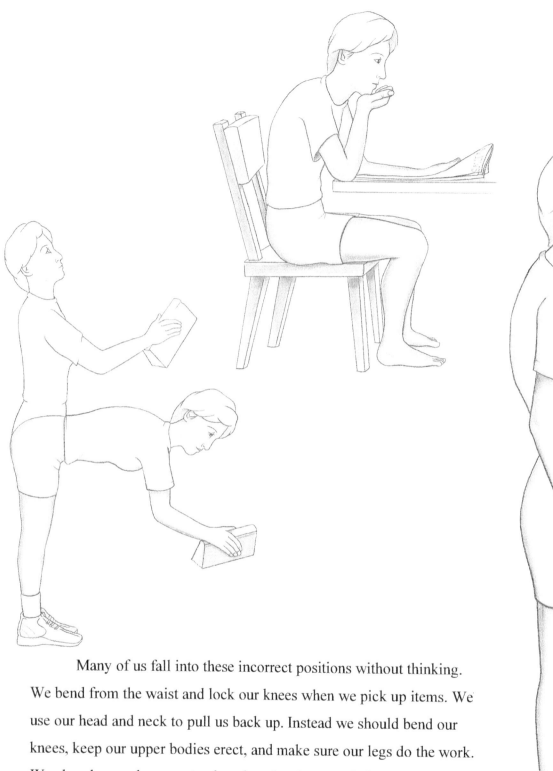

Many of us fall into these incorrect positions without thinking. We bend from the waist and lock our knees when we pick up items. We use our head and neck to pull us back up. Instead we should bend our knees, keep our upper bodies erect, and make sure our legs do the work. We also slump when we stand, and we bend our neck forward to read.

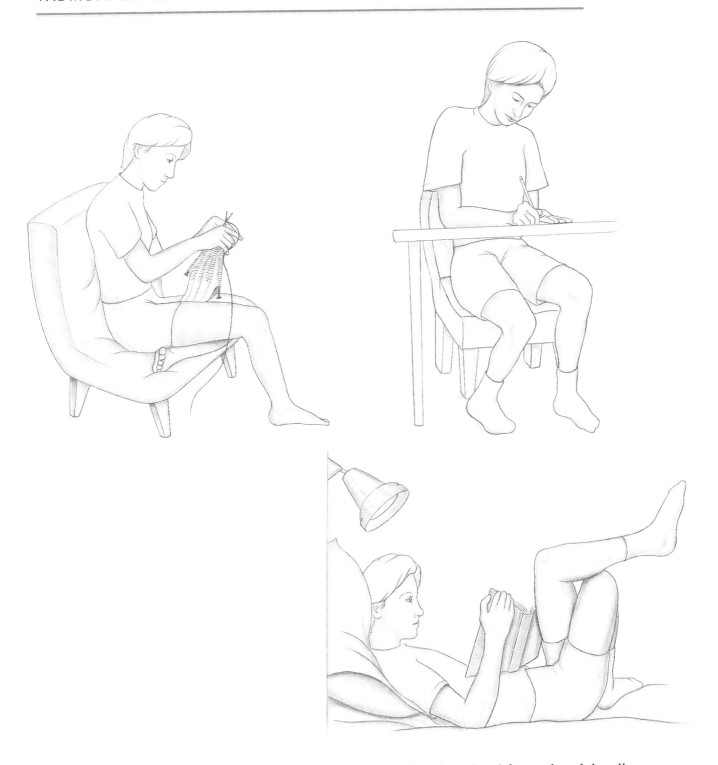

These illustrations demonstrate another common habit of continual forward neck bending. This may seem harmless or even natural, but continual irritation on the vertebrae of the neck can cause permanent damage to the nerves and spinal discs. It can cause headaches and numbness and tingling in the arms and hands with possible shoulder weakness.

STEP 2: NECK MASSAGE

You may not think of your neck as connected to pain in your arms, wrists, and fingers, but remember that everything in our bodies is connected together. The massage shown here will relax the neck muscles and increase flexibility, nerve function, and circulation.

Massage gently but firmly along both sides of the neck, using a circular motion with your fingerpads. Work down to your shoulders and back up to the skull, for one to five minutes.

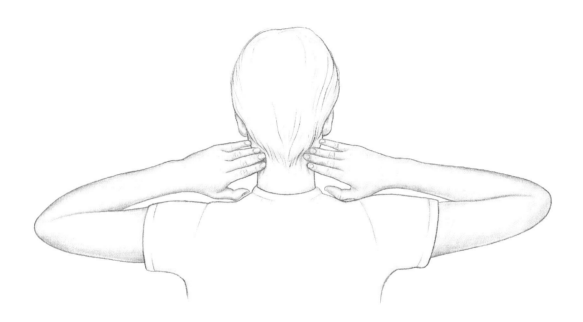

Now place your hands at the base of your skull, as shown, and gently push up with your fingers. With this traction motion, you are in essence lifting your head up off your neck and lengthening your spine. Hold for ten seconds. Remember to breathe deeply and relax.

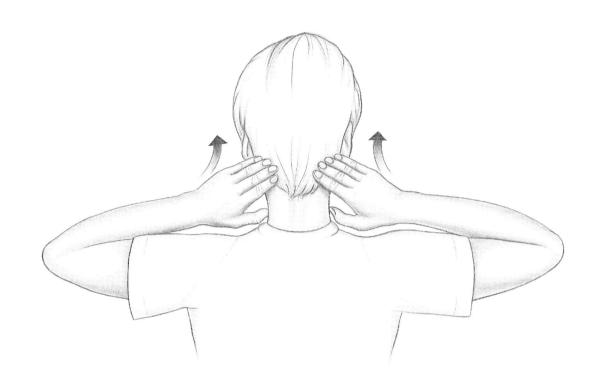

STEP 3: SHOULDER ROLLS

This exercise will relax your shoulders and upper back. Inhale and slowly roll your shoulders forward. Exhale as you move your shoulders down. Inhale and reverse the motion. Roll your shoulders backward and down as you exhale. Relax your facial muscles and breathe slowly and deeply. Roll your shoulders ten times in each direction. Repeat the exercise five to ten times in each direction.

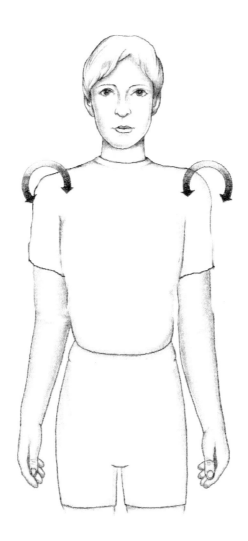

STEP 4: FORWARD ARM EXTENSION

This exercise helps realign the elbow joint in a forward line. Sometimes when your elbow joint is out of alignment and you have tendinitis, your elbow may be a bit sore after doing this exercise. Simply massage the area and the soreness will go away quickly.

With the opposite hand, palm upward, firmly support your elbow with the palm of your hand. This stabilizes the elbow joint. Then gently but firmly flick your forearm from the elbow outward as shown. Be sure to support your elbow joint. Repeat this exercise three times, first with one arm and then with the other.

Step 4 is NOT RECOMMENDED for young children.*

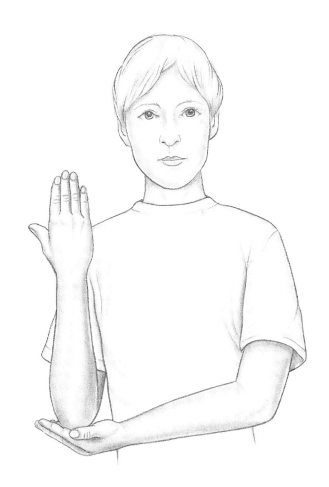

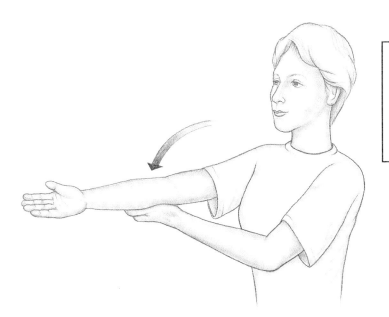

> **Important: ALWAYS SUPPORT the elbow joint, never "free-fall" the elbow joint.**
>
> *Not recommended for young children. Replace with Step 11.*

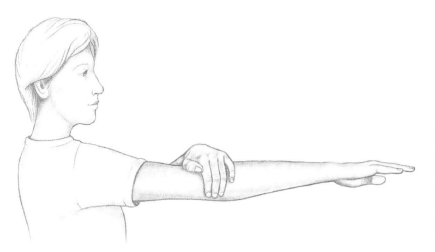

STEP 5: LATERAL ARM EXTENSION

This exercise helps realign the elbow in a lateral line. Sometimes when your elbow joint is out of alignment and you have tendinitis, your elbow may be a bit sore after doing this exercise. Simply massage the area and the soreness will go away quickly.

With your arm extended in front of you, palm down, support your elbow joint with your opposite hand. Bend your forearm to a 90-degree angle in front of your body.

Then gently but firmly flick your forearm outward as you firmly support and stabilize your elbow joint. Do not go past the shoulder line. Repeat this exercise three times, first with one arm and then with the other. Step 5 is NOT RECOMMENDED for young children.*

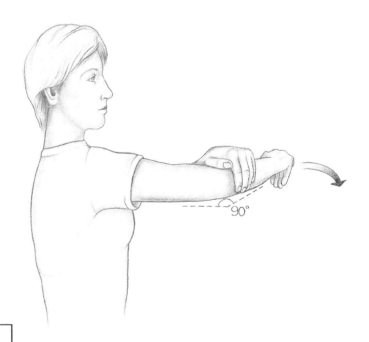

Important: ALWAYS SUPPORT the elbow joint, never "free-fall" the elbow joint.

Not recommended for young children Replace with Step 11.

STEP 6: WRIST PRESS

This exercise stretches the muscles and tendons on the front of the hand at the wrist joint.

Place your left thumb on top of your right wrist, pointing toward the elbow, and curl your fingers around the outer part of the right hand on the little finger side. This supports the right hand.

Move the supported hand as shown, flexing and extending it up and down as you press your left thumb gently but firmly into the wrist. Move your thumb slowly across the wrist, pressing into the tendons of your wrist as you continue to flex and extend it. Repeat three times, first with one wrist and then with the other.

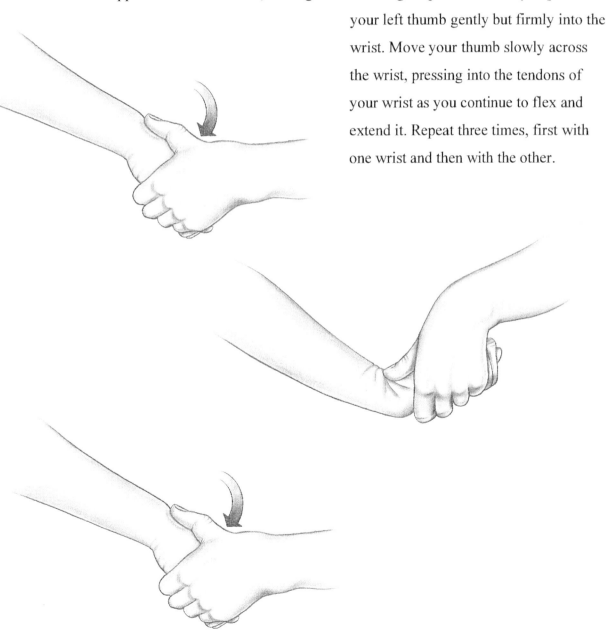

STEP 7: WRIST PULL

This exercise allows your forearm bones at the wrist to slip back into place. (You may hear the slight popping sound of the bones' shifting and realigning themselves. This is normal, so don't worry.)

Grasp the whole hand you are working on with the opposite hand. Gently but firmly pull the hand away from the wrist as shown and hold for five seconds. Repeat on your other hand.

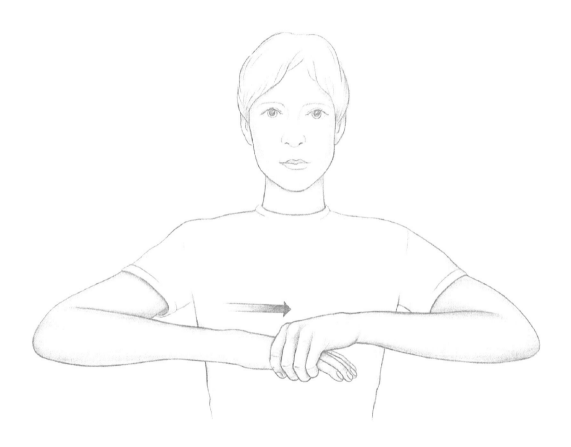

STEP 8: WRIST SQUEEZE

This exercise will help establish realignment of your wrist joint. Gently but firmly squeeze your wrist bones together. Hold for a count of two: *one-thousand-and-one, one-thousand-and-two.* Repeat on your other hand.

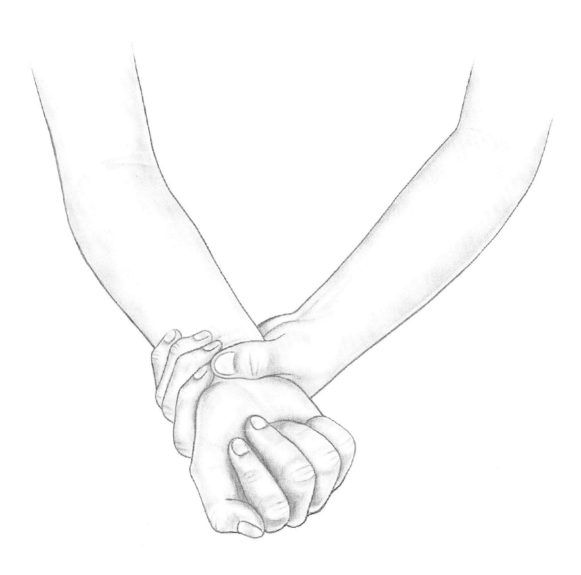

STEP 9: FINGER PULL

This exercise will help open up and restore energy within the finger joints. Again, you may hear a slight popping sound with this exercise. This is normal.

Gently grasp each finger at the base of the finger joint closest to your palm and slowly pull. Do not jerk or snap the fingers. Pull each finger once, and then repeat on the other hand. Once is enough for this exercise.

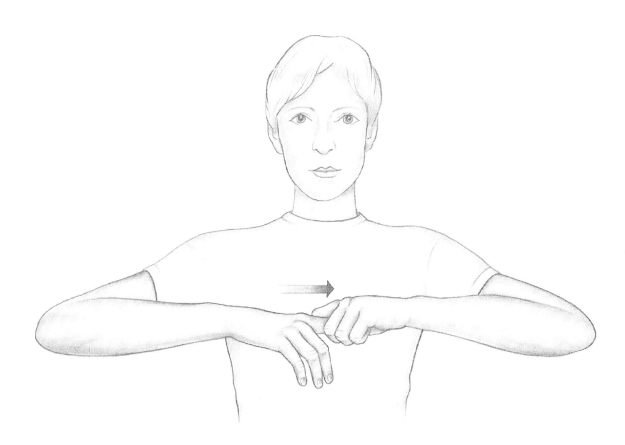

STEP 10: UPPER BACK STRETCH

This exercise feels especially good when the upper back is tired. You may stretch while you are either standing or seated.

Clasp your hands together in front of you and inhale. Exhale as you extend your arms out in front of you at chest level, stretching forward. Drop your head as shown, sink your chest inward, and round your shoulders forward. Hold this stretch for five seconds, breathing slowly and deeply (count to yourself: *one-thousand-and-one, one-thousand-and-two,* etc.). Then exhale as you release your hands and draw your shoulders back and down. Repeat this two to five times, or as often as needed.

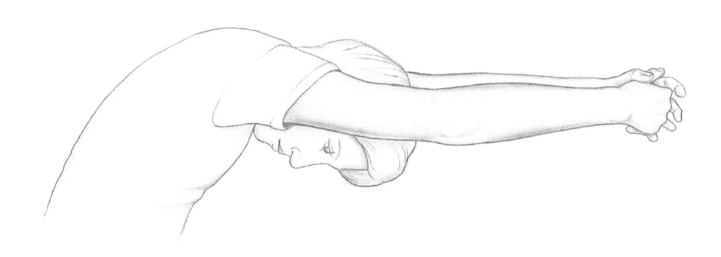

STEP 11: SHOULDER, CHEST, AND ELBOW STRETCH

This stretch can be done either sitting or standing. An added benefit is the increased nerve conductivity in the shoulder joint and the extension of the elbow joint, which helps in the realignment process.

Caution: Only stretch as far as you can comfortably. If you cannot straighten your elbows, straighten them as far as is comfortable. Every time you do the stretch, see if you can get them straighter. Eventually your chest, upper back, and arm muscles will loosen up and you will be able

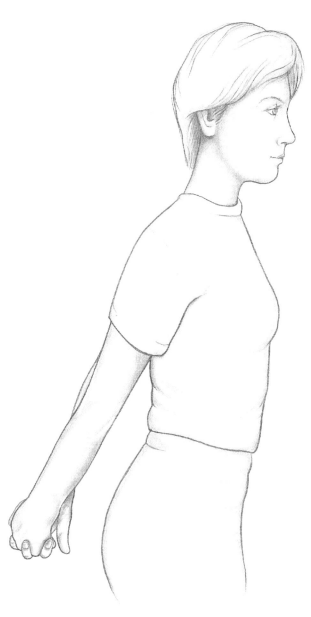

to do this stretch fully. Clasp your hands and interlace your fingers together behind your back, with your palms toward the back, and inhale. Exhale as you straighten your arms and elbows, and gently stretch your arms backwards, away from your back. Stretch slowly, and hold the stretch for five seconds. (Count to yourself: *one-thousand-and-one, one-thousand-and-two*, etc.) You can do this stretch as often as needed.

CHILDREN

Children and repetitive strain injuries are becoming just as common as adult injuries. The difference is that a child never complains and when they do, no one listens. Early prevention and maintenance is must, to avoid RSI problems in children.

Children have growing bodies that feel the strain of everyday activities just as much as an adult. Their bones while growing can also shift direction along with muscles that feel the stress of too much computer work, playing video games, participating in sports and even playing a musical instrument. It is equally as important to monitor their posture, and for school age children who are using a computer, their workstation set-up.

Ergonomics for children and young adults is another necessary step to avoid RSI problems. The workstation should accommodate your child's body. Simple as that! This alone will help your child to maintain good posture and good work habits.

The Montgomery Method, plus the programs listed in this book can be done by your child with minor changes – they are:

• For the very young child, three to five, (even babies too) massage is the most important therapy at this time. Massage can help with circulation, lymph drainage, stretching and elongation of muscles, as well as pure relaxation. Massage will remove stress and any tension and pain accumulated in their young bodies. Their muscles need continual maintenance to help with their growing body. I recently touched the arms of a five-year old drummer, and his poor arms were very tender to my touch. Massage was what he needed. All he wanted to do was play his drums, and was oblivious to any muscle discomfort.

• For the young child to young adult, six to seventeen, all twelve steps can be done with the exception of Step 4 and Step 5. It is not necessary for a child to force their elbow into alignment. A simple stretch, such as is done in Step 11, the Shoulder, Chest and Elbow Stretch, which will help to open up the shoulder and chest and help to realign the elbow joint.

Even though kids seem to have bountiful energy, they still need maintenance and regular structural alignment. Childhood RSD's are realities. The possibilities of the fullness of life require good health, and technology may rob our children of their future, both in and out of the workplace. It only makes sense to honor our children's health as much as we do our own. The International Chiropractic Pediatric Association (icpa) has a great referral system for pediatric chiropractors. Refer to the Protocol for Health in Chapter 2 for a pediatric chiropractor in your area. (Chapter 8 – Tips for children and young adults before and after using a computer or any repetitive use of the hands.)

OLDER FOLKS

Over the years I have had many older adults call me and ask me what would work for them in my book. You can do all the steps except Step 4 and Step 5. Joints that may be more brittle when we are older, arthritic, or other bone problems, and a quick snap may bring more than you bargained for. I recommend massage therapy which can help relieve tension and stress in the body as well as increase circulation, help with the elimination of waste products, pain relief and what we all need - plain old TLC. Touch deprivation is so often seen in older folks. Simple touch is what we all need to feel alive and loved. Most individuals 65+ depending on health, may have some form of arthritis, bone spurs, osteoporosis, and poor posture due to many different reasons. Before a Chiropractor or Osteopath treats you, I would recommend that you first have a x-ray examination to confirm any possible joint and spinal problems before you have an adjustment done.

The old saying that you don't want to open up a "can of worms" is very intuitive here. Your body has adapted to this posture and any major changes may disrupt body chemistry, increase pain response and arouse many variable unknowns. A Chiropractor who uses applied kinesiology (AK) techniques can help to release tension in the musculature and take stress off the spine and joints without manually adjusting your spine. (Refer to the Protocol for Health in Chapter 2 for a chiropractor that uses AK.)

Another therapy I would recommend is Crainosacral Therapy. It is very gentle, quieting to the mind, and may help release restrictions in the structure and musculature for the relief from physical discomfort. (Refer to the Resource of the book on how to locate a craniosacral practitioner in your area.)

Massage therapy is another gentle way to release tension in the muscles and keep unsettling pain and discomfort from becoming debilitating. (Refer to the Health Care Protocol in Chapter 2 for a therapist in your area)

Twelve-Step Method At A Glance

1. Posture correction
2. Neck massage
3. Shoulder rolls
4. Forward arm extension (no for children)
5. Lateral arm extension (no for children)
6. Wrist press
7. Wrist pull
8. Wrist squeeze
9. Finger pull
10. Upper back stretch
11. Shoulder, chest, and elbow stretch
12. Muscle therapy

NOW YOU'RE READY FOR STEP 12

Once you've done all these corrective techniques, reassess your perceived grip strength, as described on the previous pages. If you have a friend available, repeat the muscle monitoring test from Chapter 2 to check for muscle strength.

You can do this routine throughout your day, as often as you need to maintain structural alignment, nerve integrity, and relaxed muscles.

The next corrective technique, covered in Chapter 4, involves therapeutic muscle therapy. To relieve pain and tightness in your muscles and restore their health, flexibility, and function, you need to massage the muscles that are repeatedly overstrained and overworked. This requires a bit more time than the other steps, but you can do it before you go to work, on your lunch break, or when you get home.

Letters from...

A Technical Writer

As a technical writer, I have been suffering from RSI (repetitive strain injury) for almost a year now and have been in and out of doctor's offices, physical therapy, and tried every medication out there until I ended up with an ulcer. Kate's book is the first and only thing that I have found that works! Within 15 minutes of opening her book, I was in less pain, after 2 days, I had significantly decreased my pain, and 3 weeks later, I am finally on my way to making a recovery!

Before I started her program I was in so much pain that I could barely tie my shoes, let alone get on a computer for to work. It seemed that everything I did caused me pain and my hands even hurt when I wasn't even using them. Now, I am back on my computer, back doing what I love, and back to enjoying life again. She has really given me my life back.

Thank you, Kate'

IAN ANDERSON

Chapter 4

Muscle Therapy: The Twelfth Step

The last step of the Montgomery Method is muscle therapy, which includes four parts: trigger point release, massage therapy, myofascia stretch and release technique, and neurolymphatic massage. Using these four muscle therapy techniques, you can release pain and soreness in your muscles, strengthen your muscles and restore them to health.

After you have established structural stability by doing the first eleven steps, the next thing to do is to heal the injured muscle tissue. If this is not done, your joints will move back into the improper position they are used to, which causes a loss of nerve integrity and muscle strength. Remember: Your muscles, ligaments, and tendons hold you together, not the other way around. Muscles have a purpose, and they are feeling the pain from the overwork and overstrain of your activities. Everything has to be in balance so your body functions in harmony as it is meant to do.

Muscle therapy, accompanied by structural alignment and correct posture, is the main solution to eliminating the pain in your upper body - neck, upper back, shoulders, but most importantly, your arms and hands. Muscle therapy plays a key role in preventing carpal tunnel syndrome and other musculoskeletal injuries, and for relieving pain and avoiding surgery.

It is also therapeutic for people who have already had surgery. Thousands of people have had surgery for carpal tunnel syndrome, and many people have had multiple surgeries to try to correct this condition. People who have had surgery will have extremely sore muscles and scar tissue in the area where the surgery was performed. Before surgery, the muscles of the arms and hands were sore and tight with many trigger points. With each surgery, this situation is compounded. Muscle spasms and scar tissue can reduce movement, flexibility, and grip strength in your arms and hands and can create tremendous pain.

Muscle therapy can help restore and heal the injured tissue. Massaging the muscles of your arms and hands will release muscle spasms and dissolve and smooth out scar tissue. It also will increase circulation that will provide nutrition to heal the tissues and restore nerve function. Massage for the whole body will alleviate tightness and soreness in the muscles that support your skeletal structure. By releasing the tension in your muscles, you will feel calmer, more relaxed,

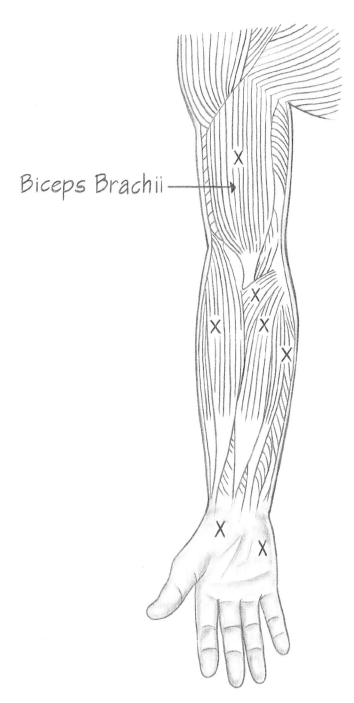

Biceps Brachii

and less stressed. With proper massage your recovery time from injury can be shortened.

The degree of muscle therapy you need is determined by your specific condition and by how many hours a day you do a repetitive task. My suggestion is to do these routines at least once a day, twice if your occupation requires you to use your hands a lot. Morning, before you begin your day and at the end of the day, to remain pain-free. You can also start your day by doing an abbreviated version of the muscle therapy program to warm up the muscles; then do the whole program at night. The massage sessions should not last more than ten minutes. When you are first getting started, you may want to consult with a qualified massage therapist if you are unable to do these routines yourself.

TRIGGER POINT RELEASE

Trigger points are hypersensitive areas in a muscle that are tender to the touch. They can be found throughout the body's musculature – in upper back, neck, shoulders, chest, arms, and hands. A trigger point may become more active when you experience physical or emotional stress or trauma. When a trigger point "fires," it sets off a continuous cycle of spasm and pain. The muscles become tighter and contract when they are overworked and overstrained, as in repetitive hand movements. The forearm and hand muscles begin to fatigue and the muscle energy in the muscle decreases. As the muscles become tighter, more and more trigger points are activated, the spasm and pain cycle intensifies, and the muscles lose mobility and refuse to work any more. The pain from a trigger point also may radiate to another area of the arm.

Self-massage for the arms and hands will help relieve tension and pain felt in your muscles because of repetitive movements. By pressing into the muscles you can locate the trigger points that cause pain in your muscles. The trigger point release and three massage strokes shown in this Chapter are easy to do and can help relieve pain in the muscles of your arms and hands.

To locate a trigger point, press into the muscle. If you feel pain, you have located a trigger point. The muscles will feel tight and ropy, and the touch of your fingertips will elicit pain. To release trigger points, hold a firm pressure in that area, up to sixty seconds or longer, and relax and breathe slowly and deeply until you feel the pain begin to subside. Then lightly massage the area and move on to another area in the muscle. The release of the trigger points, along with massage therapy described in the rest of this Chapter, will allow your muscle fibers to lengthen and relax, thereby lessening the tension and stress on the joints of the arm.

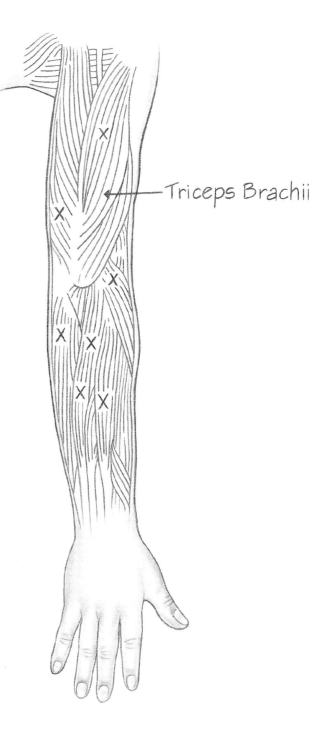

Triceps Brachii

MUSCLE THERAPY SELF-CARE

First, find a comfortable place to sit. Relax and breathe easily. Take a very small amount of a healing oil or lotion, such as arnica oil, sesame oil, jojoba, aloe lotion, or a Sports Balm. Spread it on your forearm, top and bottom, and into your hand. (You can find information on the Herbal Sports Balm later in this chapter.)

All of the following steps should be done on one arm at a time. Once you have completed muscle therapy on the first arm, move to the other arm and repeat the entire series on it.

If you have had surgery, you will want to massage that area gently but firmly, gradually working deeper. If it is painful, massage a bit more lightly. Doing this several times a day speeds the healing process and recovery time. Even if it has been many years since surgery, this therapy still works.

Muscle Therapy Strokes

There are three strokes used in working the muscles of the arms and hands: cross-fiber, broad cross-fiber, and flushing. Here's a brief explanation.

Cross-fiber: Use the pads of your fingers to press gently down into the muscle, then apply gentle but firm pressure across a muscle or tendon at a right angle. You move the muscle back and forth in a sawing motion across the muscle fibers.

Broad cross-fiber: Use your thumb to press gently but firmly into the muscle, and make a broad sweeping motion across the grain of the muscle fibers. You are still moving across the muscle grain, but in a sweeping motion rather than moving the muscle in one spot.

Flushing: This type of stroke is also called effleurage. It helps flush waste products in the muscle out through the lymphatic system. Use your forearm in long gliding strokes, always toward your heart.

Backside of the Arm and Hand

Begin on your upper forearm, palm side down, at the elbow joint. Use the cross-fiber stroke to "unweave" the painful trigger points, spasms, and knots in the muscle. With the pads of your fingers, press gently but firmly down into the muscle and move the muscle back and forth, in a sawing motion, across the muscle fibers. You will be able to feel the ropiness in your muscles. Use this stroke in small areas as you work the forearm muscles. Move down your forearm as shown, until you have done the whole arm. Repeat three times.

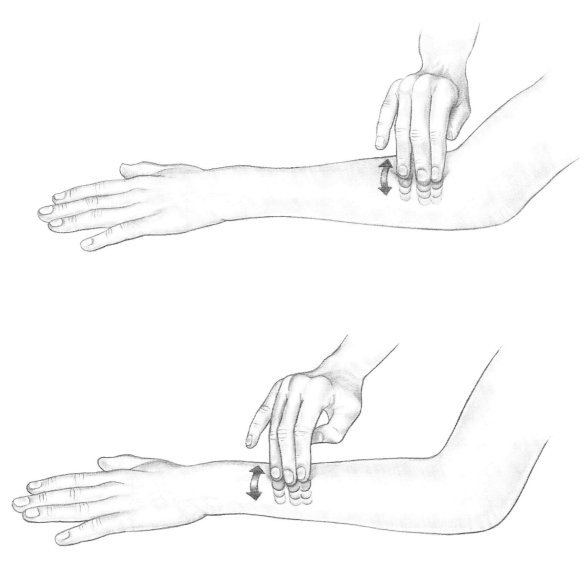

Now use the broad cross-fiber stroke to spread the fibers of the muscle to increase circulation. With your thumb, press gently but firmly into the muscle and make a broad sweeping motion across the grain of the muscle fibers. Work all the way down to the wrist and back up to your elbow three times, or as much as needed.

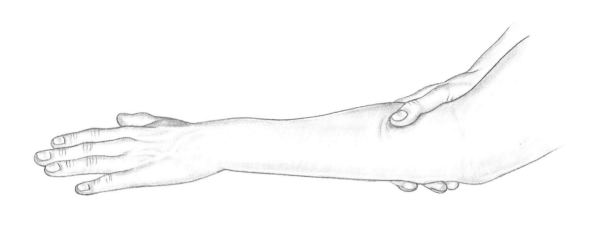

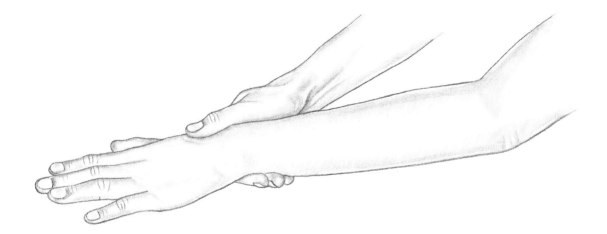

Continue by working the muscles on the top of your hand, as shown, moving into the web of your thumb and fingers. Work on the muscles as much as needed.

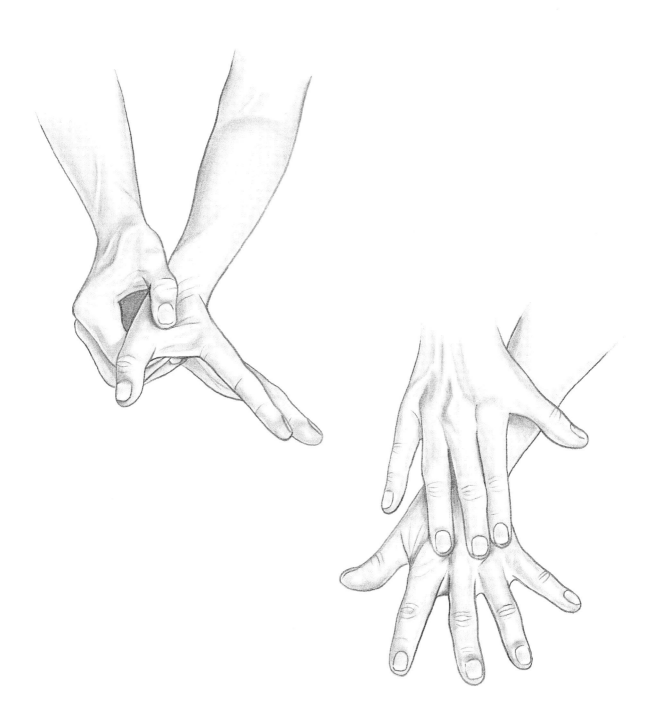

Finally, using your opposite forearm as a tool, gently but firmly press into the arm muscles and push up the forearm (toward your heart). This helps flush the waste products into the lymphatic system and out of the muscles.

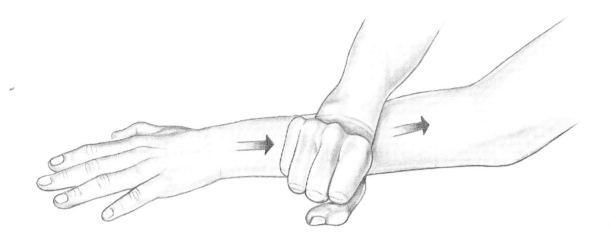

Letters from...
A Steel Guitar Player

Thanks for taking the time to show me what I was doing (wrong) and help me on the way to improved health and well-being. The well-being comes from the fact that I can again do what I love. Playing the steel guitar and entertaining was becoming a chore that my mind started aching. Now it's pure joy. I've even started playing banjo, guitar, bass, and dobro again now that my hands are no longer aching. The Montgomery Method has helped me, and I am teaching it to all my students and in seminars where I teach the steel guitar. Thanks, Kate′

JOE WRIGHT

Underside of the Arm

Begin at your elbow joint with a cross-fiber stroke. With the pads of your fingers, press firmly down into the muscle and move your fingers back and forth across the muscle fibers in a sawing motion. You will be able to feel the ropiness in your muscles. Work all the way down to your wrist. Repeat three times, or as much as needed.

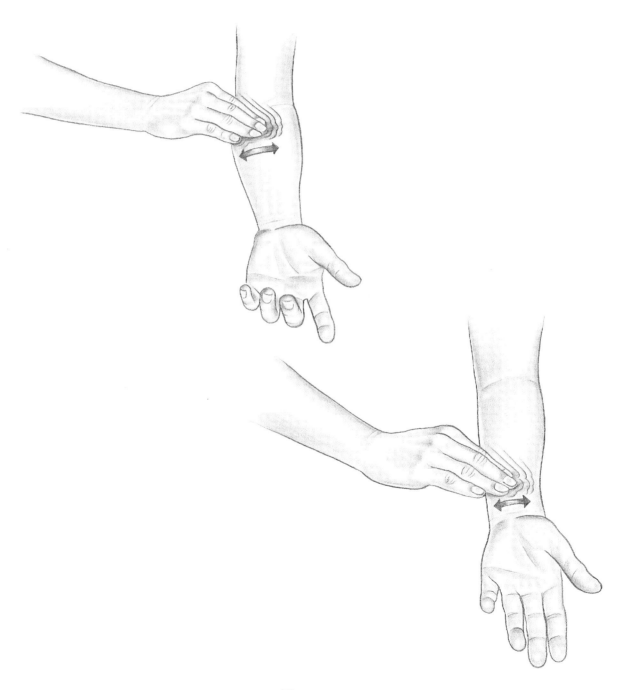

Use the broad cross-fiber stroke to spread the fibers of the muscle to increase circulation. With your thumb, press firmly into the muscle and make a broad sweeping motion across the muscles as shown below. Begin at the elbow joint, work all the way down to the wrist and then back up to the elbow. Massage your arm three times, or as much as needed.

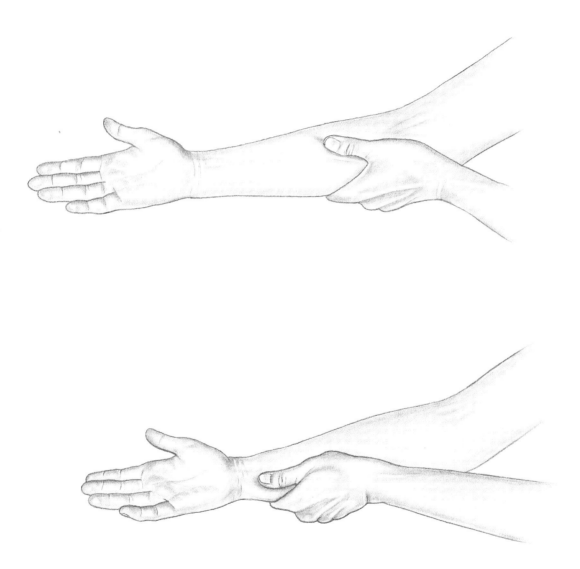

Continue to work the muscles in the palm of your hand into the pad of your thumb and fingers. Work on the muscles around the joints of the fingers and then give a gentle pull on each finger to open up the joint. Work on the hand muscles as much as needed. Remember to grasp the fingers at the point where they attach to the hand.

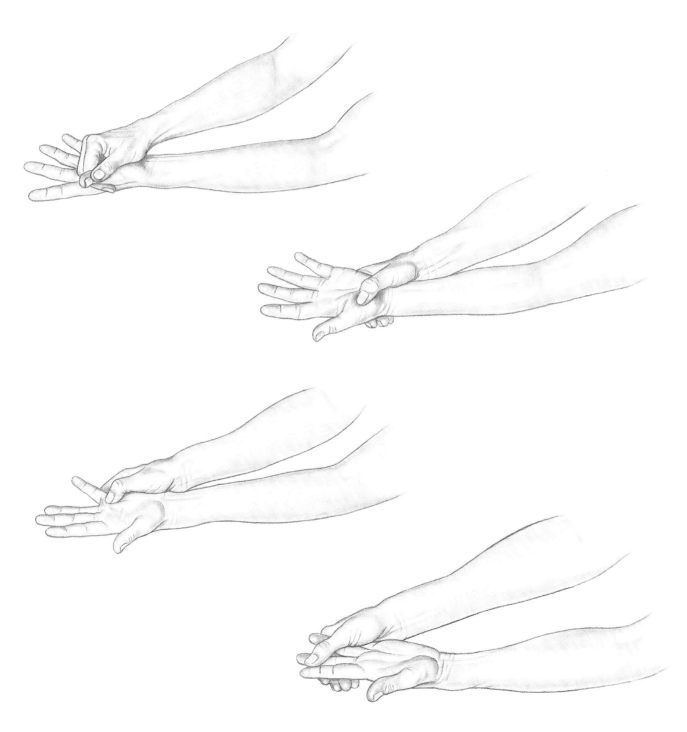

The Elbow

Many people get tendinitis or inflammation of the tendon, sometimes called tennis elbow. Massaging the tendons and muscles around the joints will help decrease the inflammation and soreness. Massage your elbow as shown below, and work the muscles in the upper arm (your triceps and your biceps). Remember to align your elbow joint – doing the forward arm extension and lateral arm extension as shown on the previous pages – which will will remove tension from your joints.

Gently massage around your elbow joints, and feel the bones of your elbow and tendon attachments. Where you feel soreness, use gentle cross-fiber and broad cross-fiber strokes.

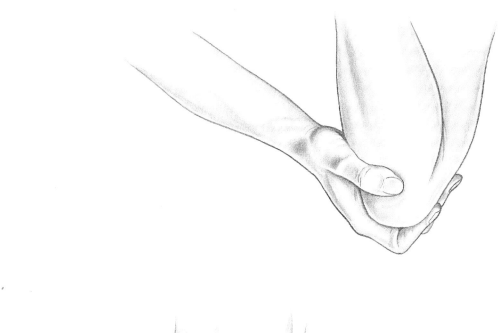

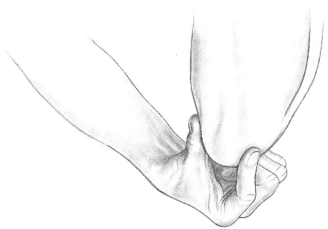

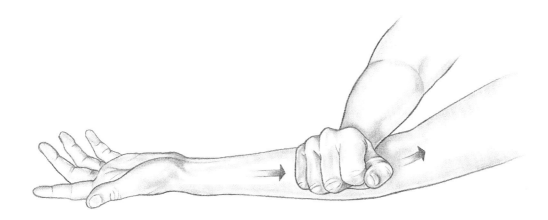

To finish, use your upper forearm as a tool to gently but firmly press into your arm muscles and press up your forearm toward your heart. This helps flush the waste products into the lymphatic system and out of the muscles. Repeat three times, or as much as needed.

Once you have completed these steps on one arm, begin again on the other arm and repeat the entire series.

MYOFASCIAL STRETCH AND RELEASE TECHNIQUE

Massage and Physical Therapists use myofascial release to help treat individuals with a variety of soft tissue problems.

What is Myofascia?

Myo is muscle and Fascia, is a thin tissue that covers every organ in the body and surrounds every muscle and every fiber within a muscle. To release the myofascia is to stretch the fascia and the muscle. "When a muscle is injured, muscle fibers tend to shorten and become tight creating unevenness within the myofascia. This unequal muscle tension can compress nerves and muscles causing pain," according to Carol J. Manheim, a physical therapist and author of *The Myofascial Release Manual*. When you press into your forearm muscles, and using a "sawing motion" you may feel "ropey" muscles and many sore spots. The ropiness is tight and shortened muscle fibers, and the sore-spots are trigger points. Injury, trauma and stress activate trigger points, and they are painful to the touch. Overuse syndromes, such as carpal tunnel and others can be helped with this technique.

BEFORE YOU BEGIN

Before you begin this technique, I recommend you hydrate your muscles by drinking a gallon of water or a quart or more of an electrolyte replacement drink, such as Gookinaid Hydralyte. Muscles tend to cramp more ready when deprived of necessary electrolytes, especially when injured. I also use a small amount of my topical Sports Balm to help begin the healing of the injured tissue. This combination has worked well for me and I have found the muscles to recovery faster with very little soreness or pain.

This technique can be done either before or after the massage. I prefer to do it after because if a person has years of overuse trauma, the pain and soreness may be too much for them to handle initially.

Remember to Breathe! Breathing will help to keep the energy moving throughout the body and lessen the pain. Always begin slowly. Use low to moderate pressure (let pain be your guide). Cover a small area of the forearm at a time. The slow movement of the opposite hand moving up and down will help to increase the release of the myofascia. As you continue to work on yourself, the tissue will slowly relax and the muscles will stretch more freely, as the pain and trigger points fade away. The improvements you are looking for are a reduction in pain to none at all, decreased muscle tension, and an increase in range of motion and flexibility. Once you have finished, massage your forearms once again. Your arms will feel light, loose, more relaxed and wonderfully alive.

STRETCH AND RELEASE OF THE EXTENSOR FOREARM MUSCLES

Position your forearm on a flat surface, palm side down, with your wrist bent, fingers pointing to the sky. Begin at the wrist. With your opposite fist, slowly but firmly press down and glide up the forearm toward the elbow as you extend the wrist, fingers pointing to the earth. Pause and rest the muscles. Allow them to "let go". Release your pressure for a moment. You will feel the tension give-way and the muscles relax. Begin again. Reposition your fist and maintain pressure. Slowly raise the hand as you continue to move up the forearm. Go a short distance, stop and rest again. Begin again lowering the hand, while you continue to maintain firm pressure on the forearm muscles, gliding upward, ending at the elbow, fingers pointing to the sky. Repeat this action one to two times or as needed.

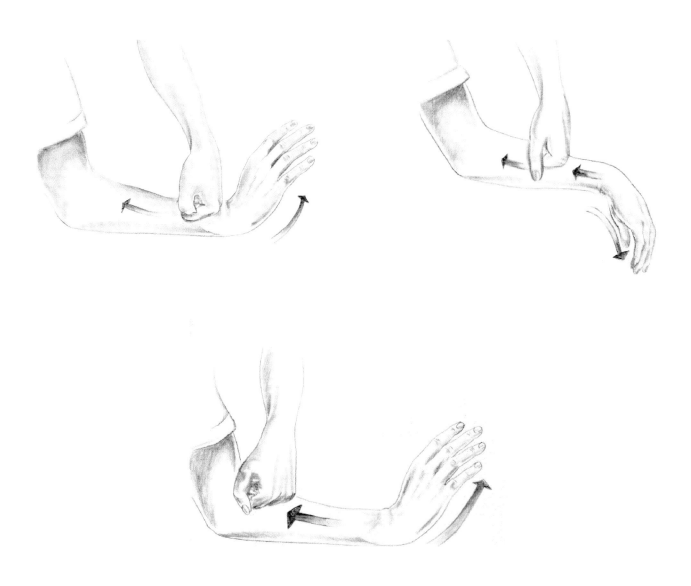

STRETCH AND RELEASE FOR THE FLEXOR FOREARM MUSCLES

Position your forearm on a flat surface, palm side up, with your wrist bent, fingers pointing to the earth. Begin at the wrist. With your opposite fist, slowly but firmly press down and glide up the forearm toward the elbow as you flex the wrist, fingers pointing to the sky. Pause and rest the muscles. Allow them to "let go". Release your pressure for a moment. You will feel the tension give-way and the muscles relax. Begin again. Reposition your fist and maintain pressure. Slowly lower the hand as you continue to move up the forearm. Go a short distance, stop and rest again. Begin again and raise the hand, while you continue to maintain firm pressure on the forearm muscles, gliding upward, ending at the elbow, fingers pointing to the earth. Repeat this action one to two times or as needed.

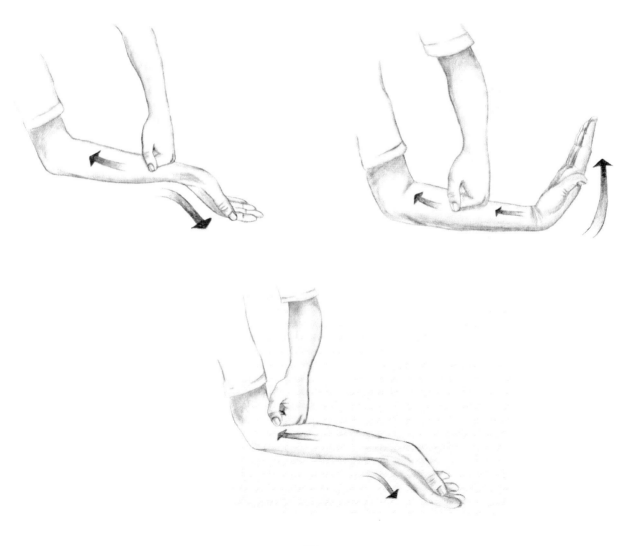

THE LYMPHATIC SYSTEM

The lymphatic system is the cleansing system of the body. It plays a pivotal role in the body's defense mechanism against disease. It helps filter out and dispose of metabolic waste products, toxins, and bacteria that accumulate in the body.

The lymphatic system is composed of nodes that are made up of a network of vessels, capillaries, and ducts. Our lymphatic system produces disease-fighting cells known as lymphocytes, and the system is continuously detoxifying the body and strengthening the immune system.

When we do repetitive movements with our muscles, we are exercising. When our arm and hand muscles are constantly moving, they are accumulating metabolic waste products that make our muscles feel sore, heavy, and fatigued. Our lymph system is constantly flushing our muscles, but some times it takes days before our muscles feel better. Neurolymphatic massage will speed up this process.

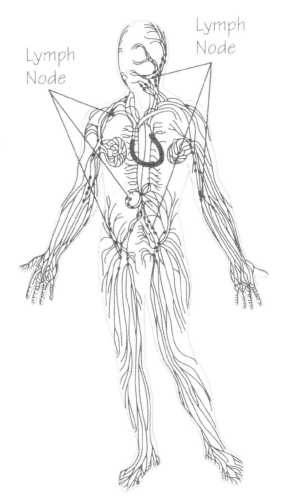

To address the pain associated with carpal tunnel, you also have to address problems in the muscles and ligaments linked to your wrist and hand. I use applied kinesiology, which is the study of muscle activity, to detect imbalances. An applied kinesiologist might stimulate or relax muscles to eliminate health problems. Within this system there are neurolymphatic reflex points called the Chapman reflexes. Frank Chapman, D.O. discovered the neurolymphatic reflex points in the 1930s and correlated them with specific glands and organs. In the 1960s George Goodheart, D.C. correlated the Chapman reflexes with specific muscles.

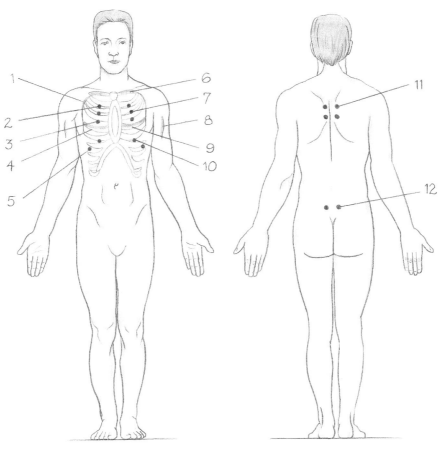

1. Supraspinatus
2. Subscapularis
3. Pronator Teres
4. Pectoralis Sternal and Rhomboids
   (this point is on the right side only)
5. Latissimus Dorsi, Triceps, Middle
   and Lower Trapezius, Hand
6. Neck Flexors and Extensors

7. Deltoid
8. Upper Trapezius
9. Pectoralis Clavicular and Brachioradialis
   (this point is on the left side only)
10. Biceps, Supinator, Hands
11. Deltoid
12. Hand Muscles

All points except 4 and 9 are on both sides of the body

Rubbing the neurolymphatic reflex points will detoxify and enhance the function of your organs, glands, and muscles while strengthening your immune system. There is a close relationship between your muscles and your organs and glands. In my program, we work primarily on the muscles. The specific points and areas that affect the upper body muscles are shown in the illustration above. Every muscle has an associated neurolymphatic reflex point. Rubbing these points firmly and deeply alleviates the pain and soreness by decreasing the inflammation.

There are two types of muscles: healthy and unhealthy. An unhealthy muscle that is overworked and overstrained will feel sore, tight, and painful to the touch. A healthy muscle will feel light, relaxed, flexible, supple, and free of pain.

Locate the specific point or mark on the diagram. Press or rub firmly but gently for thirty seconds to five minutes or until the pain, soreness, and inflammation have decreased in the affected muscle and it feels light and more mobile. Rub points as often as needed, using a firm but gentle pressure.

These techniques can also be used to help your muscles recover from sports activities such as golf, tennis, handball, and rowing.

KATE'S SPORTS BALM

Through research and experience and with the help of my dear friend, herbalist John Finch, we created a product that we believe helps heal injured soft tissue. We call this Sports

---

What's in the Sports Balm

Here's what Sports Balm includes and what each ingredient does:

- black walnut leaves: astringent
- chaparral: antiseptic
- comfrey leaf and root: demulcent, vulnerary, astringent
- lobelia: antispasmodic
- marshmallow:, demulcent, emollient, vulnerary
- mullein leaf: astringent, vulnerary, demulcent
- skullcap: antispasmodic
- white oak bark: astringent
- wormwood: antiseptic
- gravel root: astringent, antiseptic, demulcent

An antiseptic inhibits growth of microorganisms; an antispasmodic prevents or eases muscular spasm or convulsions; an astringent contracts tissues and slows the discharge of fluid; a demulcent soothes inflamed surfaces and protects them from irritation; an emollient softens tissues; and a vulnerary promotes cell growth and wound healing.

Balm, or Herbal Healing Balm. It is an all-natural, organic, wild-crafted herbal mixture with the scent of wintergreen extracted from ten herbs and eleven other ingredients that help heal injured tissue. It is safe to use with homeopathic medicines. We use it for the relief of sprains, strains, aching and swollen joints, bruising, muscle soreness and adhesions. It can even be used on cuts and scrapes, without scarring. You need only use a small amount, as it goes a long way.

Letters from...

A Harpist

If you can imagine a whole year of dealing with increasing pain, being able to do less and less, and terribly anxious about not being able to continue my career in music – the relief and the new hope that this pain-free state engendered were very dramatic. I felt overwhelmed with gratitude toward this knowledgeable woman. I have learned the reasons for the pain, and that knowledge has strengthened my resolve to take the corrective healing measures that Kate has taught me. It all makes sense-and Kate is showing me the way!

SHEILA STERLING, PRINCIPAL HARPIST
SAN DIEGO SYMPHONY AND SAN DIEGO OPERA

You can use it not only during your regular daily muscle therapy, but also to help heal the injured tissue of strains, sore muscles, sprains, even open cuts and abrasions. Rub on a small amount of Sports Balm. If your hands are too tired or sore to work on the muscles, place a medium hot cloth compress, cotton is best-over the area. To insulate and keep the heat in, wrap a plastic bag around the cloth, and then add another towel. Use a heating pad if you have one, but take care not to fall asleep with a heating pad turned on (it can burn you severely). Sit for thirty minutes. The Sports Balm will penetrate into your muscles, relieving your soreness, increasing healing, and decreasing recovery time. Your muscles will feel great the next day.

If you have an injured ankle, rub Sports Balm all over the injured area, and after an hour begin range-of-motion exercises and micro-movements of the ankle. The objective is to increase mobility without pain and to prevent the formation of scar tissue. Repeat the hot compresses and reapply Sports Balm as often as possible in the first twenty-four hours of an injury. While most sports doctors will tell you to use ice to prevent inflammation in the first twenty-four hours – the routine known as Rest, Ice, Compression,

Elevation (RICE) – we have found this combination of herbs and heat when used together to be very effective in decreasing recovery time.

Once the swelling has gone down, gently massage the muscles using a broad cross-fiber stroke. This increases the blood supply to heal the soft tissue and flush waste products out of the lymphatic system.

To order the Sports Balm, order on-line at:

Web: http:// www.sportstouch.com

Email: orders@sportstouch.com

Chapter 5

Relieve Your Pain Through Acupressure

Once you have finished working on your muscles, you have one more important thing to do to speed healing and maintain health. This next step is using acupressure, a way of healing by pressing specific points on your body. Acupressure is a safe and noninvasive form of therapy that helps relieve pain and muscle soreness and decreases muscle inflammation.

According to traditional Chinese theory, pain and soreness indicate an imbalance in energy pathways. These energy pathways are called meridians. Each meridian is associated with an organ system or extra energy pathway located throughout the body.

Acupressure points are places on the skin that are hypersensitive. The acupressure points in this Chapter are the same points used in the Chinese system of acupuncture. By pressing on acupressure points, you can release blocked energy that can then flow throughout the body to relieve pain and muscle soreness. Both healing methods have been used for thousands of years. By pressing these specific points, you can restore vital energy, strength, circulation, and balance as well as relieve pain. The area benefits from increased blood flow and oxygen, helping the muscles to relax and heal. Acupressure also relieves tension and helps your body resist illness. Some doctors theorize that this pressure stimulates the nervous system to release endorphins, which can relieve pain and affect mood.

You can assess your pain level and apply pressure to these points as often as you feel the need. Acupressure is a preventive technique to ensure a healthier and more relaxed body, and it can help your immune system recover.

You will probably want to wear the most comfortable clothing possible, as tight clothing can interfere with your circulation and breathing. It's best to wash your hands thoroughly before beginning, especially before touching any points near the eyes.

POINT 1: LARGE INTESTINE 4

Arm, hand, and finger pain

Pressure at this point will relieve contracture and pain in your arms, hands, and fingers and will relieve pain from strains and sprains.

Warning: It is recommended that pregnant women do not use this point, as it might cause contractions.

Locate the point in the middle of the web between your thumb and second finger. Press and rub firmly for ten to thirty seconds or as long as needed to achieve results. Relax and breathe slowly and deeply. Repeat on the opposite hand.

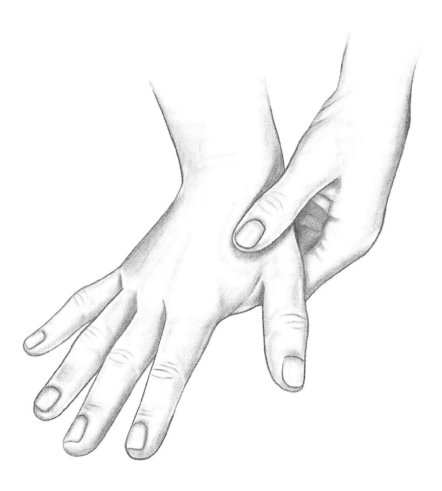

POINT 2: BAXIE POINTS

Spasms in hand muscles

Pressure at these points will relieve spasms and contracture in the hand muscles and increase circulation and decrease swelling.

Locate points on the top of your hand, between the knuckles, at the beginning of the fingers. Press and rub firmly for ten to thirty seconds or as long as needed to achieve desired results. Relax and breathe slowly and deeply. Repeat on the opposite hand.

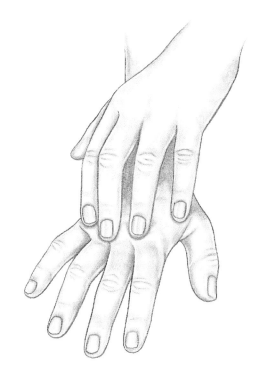

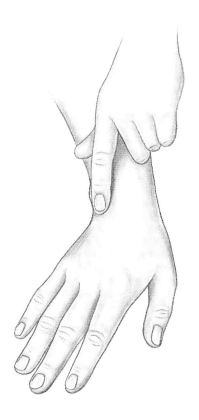

POINT 3: TRIPLE WARMER 4

Shoulder, arm, wrist, and hand pain

Pressure at this point increases energy, relieves shoulder, arm, wrist, and hand pain.

Locate the point on the top of the hand, little finger side, in the crease of the wrist in the front of the ulna bone (this bone sticks up slightly). Place your thumb on the middle of your wrist crease, with your fingers on the inside of your wrist. With your thumb and finger or knuckles, gradually apply firm pressure to the hollow spaces between the bones. Press firmly for ten to thirty seconds, or as long as needed to achieve pain relief. Relax and breathe slowly and deeply. Repeat on the opposite hand.

POINT 4: PERICARIUM 6

Elbow and arm pain and contracture

Pressure at this point will help relieve pain and muscle contracture in the elbow and arm. It can also relieve nausea and anxiety.

Locate the point on the inside of the forearm, a bit more than two fingers' width from the

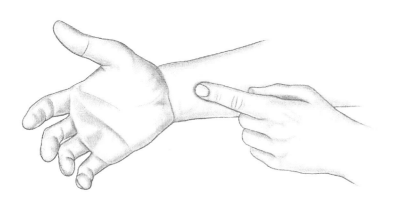

crease of the wrist, in the center of the forearm between the tendons. Press firmly for ten to thirty seconds or as long as needed. Relax and breathe slowly and deeply. Repeat on the opposite hand.

POINT 5: HEART 7

Relaxing your arm muscles

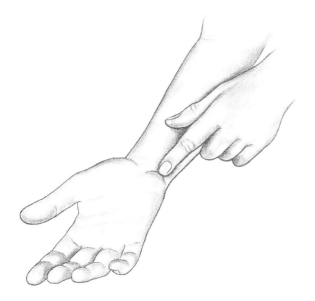

Pressure at this point will help relax the muscles of your arms as well as the rest of your body. It can also help relieve anxiety.

Locate the point on the inside of your forearm – the little finger side – in the crease of your wrist at the junction of your wrist and hand. Press and hold lightly. Gently massage. Breathe slowly and deeply. Hold as long as needed. Repeat on the opposite hand.

POINT 6: GALLBLADDER 1

Headaches, failing vision, eye redness

This point will help relieve headaches, failing vision, and eye redness.

Locate the point in the depression at the lateral side of the eye socket, as shown. Press and rub gently but firmly for ten to thirty seconds or as long as needed to achieve desired results. Close your eyes, relax, and breathe deeply. (Press and rub the corresponding point on the opposite side of the face at the same time for maximum relief.)

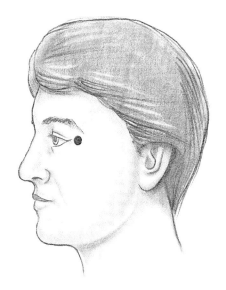

POINT 7: GALLBLADDER 14

Headaches, blurry vision, eye pain

This point will help relieve headaches, blurry vision, and pain in the eye.

Locate the points on the forehead as shown, one finger's width above and roughly in the middle of each eyebrow. Press and rub gently but firmly for ten to thirty seconds or as long as needed for desired relief. Close your eyes, relax, and breathe deeply.

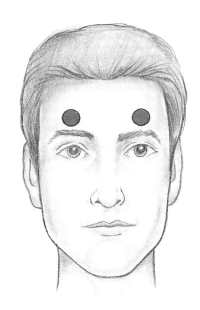

POINT 8: GALLBLADDER 37

Clearer Vision

This point helps you have clearer vision.

Locate the point on the outside of your lower leg, in the middle, one-third of the way up, above the ankle bone. Press and rub gently but firmly for ten to thirty seconds or as long as needed for relief. Close your eyes, relax, and breathe deeply. Repeat on the opposite leg.

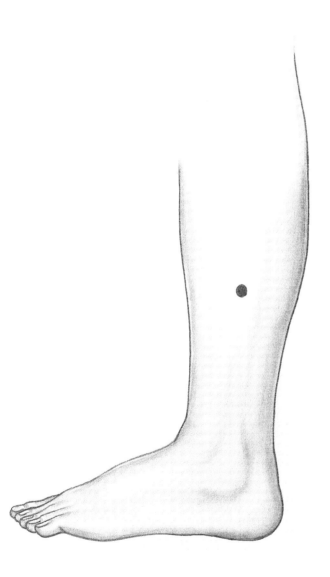

POINT 9: BLADDER 1 OR EYEBRIGHT

Eye swelling, redness, and pain

Pressure at this point can help relieve eye swelling, redness, and pain of the eye.

Close your eyes. Locate the points at the inside corners of your eyes, in the hollow. Press gently with medium pressure. (Use special care if you wear contact lenses.) Hold for ten to thirty seconds. Close your eyes, relax, and breathe deeply.

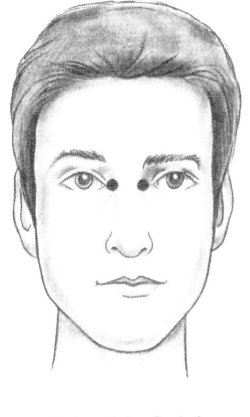

POINT 10: BLADDER 2

Headaches and eye pain, swelling, blurry vision

Pressure at this point will help relieve headaches, pain and swelling of the eye, and blurry vision.

Locate the points at the inside ends of your eyebrows. Press and rub gently but firmly for ten to thirty seconds or as long as needed for relief. Relax and breathe deeply.

RELAXING YOUR MUSCLES

After you have pressed and held the points, massage the temples, forehead, and muscles around the eyes using light pressure with your fingertips and applying small circular motions. Relax and breathe deeply. You can complete this with the relaxation palming technique. To do this, rub your palms together briskly, then put them lightly over your eyes. The warmth from your hands will help your eye muscles relax.

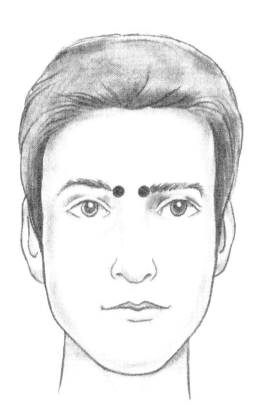

Breathing is the Rhythm of Life It Gives you Energy and your Health:

Breathing for Better Health and Energy

When we are born, we naturally breathe correctly, deeply, and from the abdomen, using the diaphragm muscle. When we get older, however, we tend to adopt incorrect breathing habits.

Breathing correctly can increase your lung volume and help you get more oxygen to your muscles and other body tissues. Breathing too shallow; however, can upset the pH balance of the blood and can prevent sufficient oxygen from reaching your muscles. It can also cause a decrease in the flow of calcium into the tissues, which can cause hypersensitive muscles. In turn, this can make you nervous or anxious and cause feelings of confusion.

Breathing only from the chest area does not allow for the correct use of the diaphragm muscle used in normal breathing and to allow you to take in a fuller, deeper breath. When we become teenagers and into adulthood, we watch TV, read ads about having a smaller waistline. This suggest to us to "suck in" our abdominal muscles and keep them there. This totally negates the use of the diaphragm muscle.

Instead, you need to learn to breathe from your diaphragm, which expands up into the whole chest cavity, raises the shoulder girdle and extends the neck muscles. The health benefits of diaphragmatic breathing increases oxygen throughout your body and into your brain. This will make you feel calmer, sharpen your memory, and give you more energy, better coordination, better stamina, and endurance to complete your tasks at hand. It allows you to focus and to become fully present in your body. Your awareness is sharpened and mental acuity is enhanced.

Our lungs are made of tiny tubes called bronchioles. At the end of these tubes are tiny air sacs called alveoli. These sacs are like little balloons, waiting to be inflated with oxygen to help distribute oxygen into our blood and to move it into our muscles, organs, and brain. When this doesn't work well, it leaves us fatigued, short of breath, and run down.

Retraining yourself to diaphragmatically breathe once again, takes practice. This is how to begin: Find a quiet place to lie down. Prop a pillow under your knees, and your neck if desired. Close your eyes. Place your hands on your upper abdomen, just below your rib cage, and focus on this area. As you inhale, push your abdomen outward, and as your breath deepens, feel the air rise up into your chest, then to your shoulder area, and further up, as you feel your neck muscles extend. Hold for a slight second, then exhale slowly and begin again.

As you move the air up, starting from the abdominal area. your abdomen protrudes. As the air rises, you may feel a "catch- when the air doesn't go where you want it to. These catches will disappear as you become accustomed to breathing from the diaphragm. Learning how to breathe from your diaphragm may feel awkward at first. Keep practicing! It will become easier with each breath you take.

Chapter 6

Stretching, Strengthening, and Range-of-Motion Exercises

Maintenance is the Key to Prevention!

When you have followed the program in this book consistently, you will achieve structural and muscular balance. To remain pain-free and stay aligned, however, you should follow the following steps for best results from the Montgomery Method.

How will you know when you are ready for these maintenance exercises?

There are two ways to confirm that you are ready to do the maintenance routines. First, you will feel a difference in your own body. Your pain will lessen or disappear. You will be comfortable doing your work and hobbies. Second, your health practitioner – whether you have chosen a chiropractor, acupuncturist, or physician – will determine if you are structurally and muscularly in balance.

> *Please remember: Until you are structurally and muscularly balanced,*
> *and nerve pain, numbness and tingling has left, and you are pain free,*
> *(not the muscle pain from exercise), then you can begin a sound program*
> *for stretching and strengthening.*

When and where you do these exercises is up to you. Find a time and place that is convenient for you. Consistency is the most important aspect. Do the exercises as often as needed to be comfortable.

> **If you do not maintain your corrected alignment, your symptoms will return.**
> **If you do not follow a regular massage schedule, then your muscles will**
> **develop trigger points and pain will return.**

ROUTINES TO MAINTAIN PROPER ALIGNMENT

Stretching, strengthening, and range-of-motion exercises are essential to maintain the flexibility, mobility, and strength of your body. A daily routine, once your body has been brought back into balance by the methods outlined earlier, will help you stay focused and in control of how your body feels.

Your goal is to be pain-free. The body is not meant to be in pain. The benefits of these types of programs have been covered in many books and articles and are well known and accepted.

Your goals for stretching are to:

- increase your flexibility and range of motion
- reduce stress and tension in your muscles
- reduce chance of injuries
- gain a sense of well-being and alertness that lasts throughout the entire day.

If you want to maintain your recovery, you need a consistent maintenance program. You cannot follow a program for a couple of months and then start sitting around again. If you cease these exercises and follow a sedentary lifestyle, your carpal tunnel pain will return.

WHY YOU WANT TO WARM UP

Never hit the floor running. This is the same advice I give the athletes I work with. Every person should prepare the body to perform a job, no matter what it is. For a physical task, you should warm up the body. Beginning cold without a proper warm-up can cause an injury.

Warm up for five to ten minutes to increase circulation in your muscles. Pump them up! Do twenty or so jumping jacks or march in place for five minutes to warm up your body. Do range-of motion exercises for the shoulders, arms, and hands. These include arm circles, shoulder rolls, shoulder shrugs, reach-for-the-sky stretches, and side bends. Anything you can do to increase your shoulder and upper body flexibility will help prevent musculoskeletal disorders.

Stretch for ten to fifteen minutes before you start your workday. Here are some rules to remember while stretching:

- Never stretch cold. Warm up first
- Never bounce or force a stretch
- Try to keep the body in alignment when stretching
- Remember to breathe and relax into the stretch.

HINTS FOR STRETCHES AND EXERCISES

Do these slowly and gently. Only stretch as far as your body will allow you. Never force a stretch. In time, your flexibility and range of motion will increase as you continue to do stretches. Hold each one at least one minute. Do not rush through a stretch, as this defeats the purpose. Remember to breathe.

You can do these stretches in the morning, at break time, and at the end of your day. Remember, just a few minutes of stretching done throughout your day can help prevent injuries. Of course, if you feel you cannot do a stretch, listen to your body and do not do it. Your body will be different on different days. Do not give up on a stretch; keep trying it, and eventually it will feel right for your body.

After stretching, rub the neurolymphatic points shown in Chapter 5. This will help your muscles remain energetically strong and more relaxed. All these exercises and stretches should be done slowly and with concentration. When strengthening the ligaments and tendons, use light weights – no more than one or two pounds. While the goal is to first strengthen the ligaments and tendons that hold the joints together, the muscles will also strengthen and tone.

Letters from...
An Administrative Secretary

I had surgery for carpal tunnel syndrome but still had tremendous pain in the wrist, arm, and elbow. Kate' has taught me self-correcting techniques to relieve the stress and tension by realigning the wrist and elbow, which I can do as needed, diminishing the pain, enabling me to get through the day and do my job. As a result of Kate's massage therapy and pain relief training, I will not undergo surgery on my elbow or on my other wrist. There are not enough words in the human language to express my gratitude. I only wish I had found you sooner.

CYNTHIA WEAVER

Don't overdo the exercises. The goal is to be able to do three sets of each exercise without feeling pain or soreness. If your wrists are sore after the second set of ten, stop. A slow building-up period of two to three months, using only light weights, will strengthen your ligaments and tendons. Stay consistent and the results will show.

Letters from...

A Legal Secretary

I've been employed as a legal secretary for the past twelve years. A month ago I began experiencing stiffness and pain in my left hand. Eventually the pain was radiating into my elbow all the way up to my left shoulder and my neck. By the end of the day, 1 was in tears with pain.

I went to an orthopedic physician who, on the first visit, suggested surgery. I was wearing a splint on my left hand and a few weeks later my right hand began to tingle and feel numb. The pain was bad, but it was extremely frustrating for me because 1 couldn't hold a newspaper, fold clothes, work in the garden. or do anything that required the use of my hands. The frustration alone was beginning to persuade me to have surgery. A friend gave me Kate's book.

That night. I began to do some of the exercises illustrated in your book. First, my elbow popped and there was an incredible release of the pain. Next, my fingers popped. I just looked at my hands with amazement. I can't believe how fast the results happened.

This happened just last night, and today I'm writing this letter without any pain, fatigue, or stiffness. Yesterday morning I couldn't even write a sentence without having to put down the pen in frustration from the pain.

You don't have to get surgery for carpal tunnel syndrome. I'm living proof.

– DEBBIE HARNOIS

STRETCHING EXERCISES FOR THE NECK

Checking range of motion

To check for range of motion of the neck, first turn your head to the right, and then to the left. Feel the difference in muscle tightness between the two sides. (After you have done the exercises for the shoulder and neck, which are described in detail in this Chapter, repeat this exercise to see if your range of motion has improved and if the tightness in your neck and shoulders has decreased.)

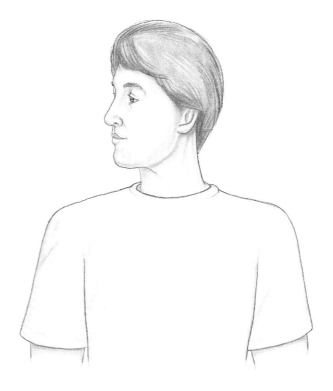

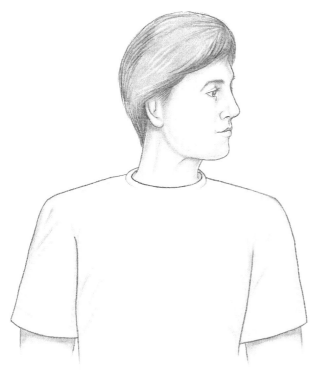

Neck release

To help release tension in your neck muscles, place your hand, palm down, over the back of your neck on one side as shown below. Firmly press the pads of your fingers along the edge of the neck vertebrae and squeeze the neck muscles. Maintain firm pressure as you move your head forward and back. Do this exercise slowly, ten times. Relax and breathe slowly and deeply. Repeat this exercise on the opposite side of your neck.

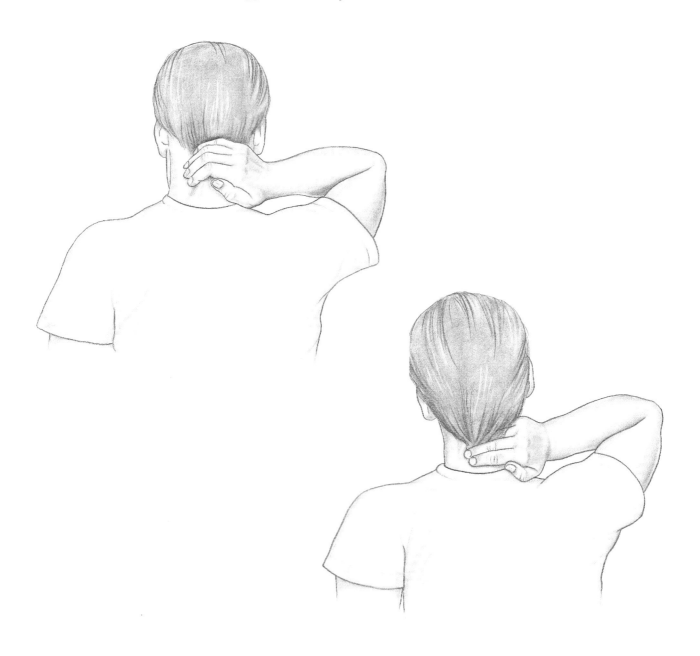

Isometric stretch

Isometric exercises done throughout your range of motion – moving your head forward, backward, and to each side – help strengthen and stretch the muscles, tendons, and ligaments of your neck.

Place your hand on the side of your head as shown. Inhale, and then as you exhale, gently push into your hand with approximately two (2) percent of your strength for a five-second count. Release. Slowly stretch your neck a little farther. Repeat the stretch three times in each direction, as shown both sides, forward and back. *Do not pull on neck; stretch only as far as is comfortable.*

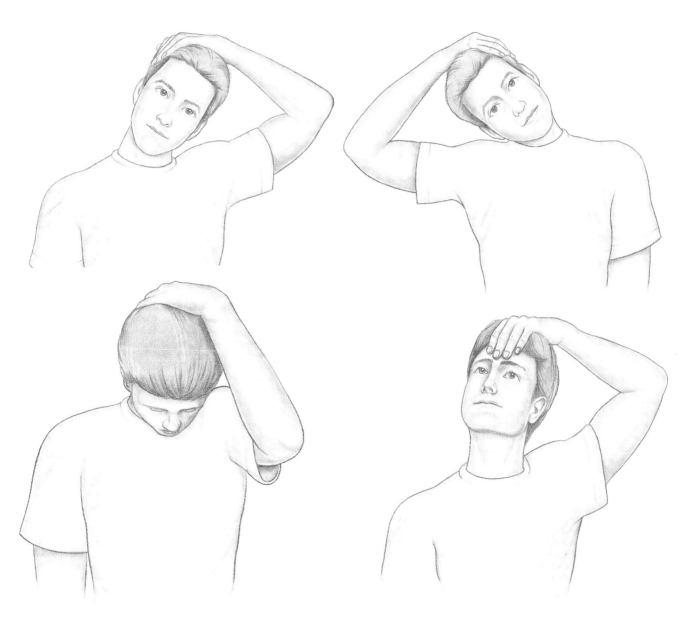

RANGE-OF-MOTION EXERCISES FOR THE SHOULDER

These exercises help release tension in the shoulder muscles and increase their range of motion.

Shoulder half-circles

This helps release tension in your shoulder muscles and increases your range of motion. While standing or sitting, bend your elbow to ninety degrees as shown and hold it close to your body. With your opposite hand, firmly grasp your upper shoulder muscle as you move your arm forward and backward slowly for ten half-circles. Maintain firm pressure at all times throughout the movement, pinching the shoulder muscle as you relax and breathe slowly and deeply. Repeat on the other shoulder, ten times. Repeat this exercise as often as needed.

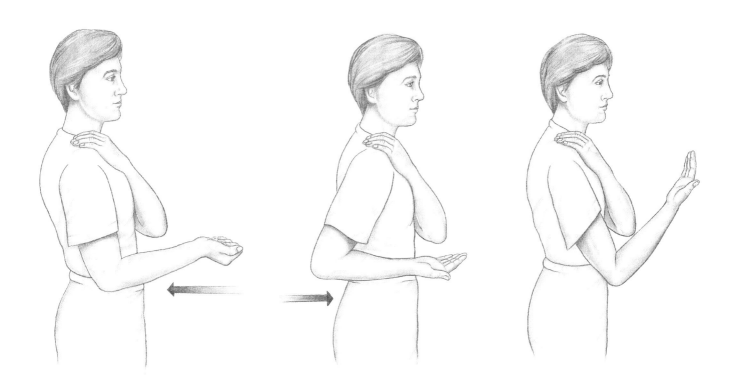

Shoulder raises full-circles

This helps release tension in your shoulder muscles and increases your range of motion. While standing or sitting, bend your elbow and raise your arm to shoulder level. With your opposite hand, firmly grasp your upper shoulder muscle. Maintain firm pressure, pinching the muscle as you move your arm slowly in a clockwise direction ten times. Continue to hold pressure on your shoulder muscle, relax, and breathe slowly and deeply. Repeat with the other shoulder in a counterclockwise direction, also for ten times. Repeat as often as needed.

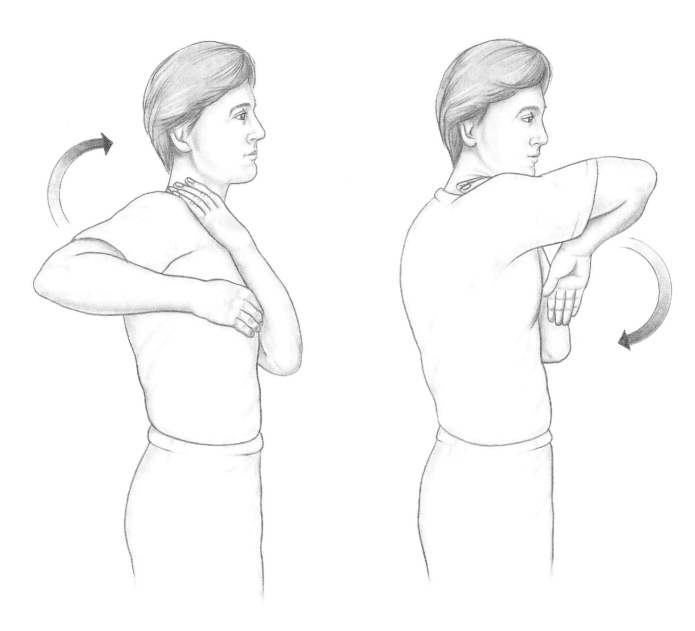

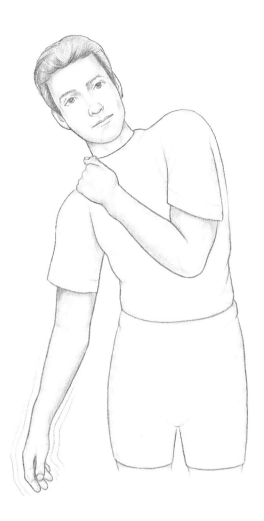

Shoulder shakes

This helps relax the shoulder muscles. Raise one hand to your opposite shoulder and grasp the shoulder muscle. Lean over to the side and shake your arm that is hanging down. Hold firm pressure on your shoulder muscle for ten seconds. Relax and breathe slowly and deeply. Repeat on the other shoulder as much as needed.

Shoulder shrugs

This exercise will relax your shoulders and upper back. Inhale as you slowly raise your shoulders to your ears. Hold for a five-second count. Exhale and slowly lower your shoulders. Breathe slowly and deeply. Repeat these shrugs ten times.

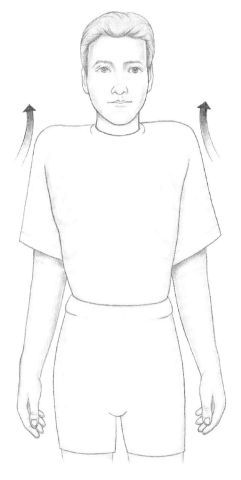

Shoulder rolls

This exercise will relax your shoulders and upper back. Inhale and slowly roll your shoulders forward. Exhale as you move your shoulders down. Inhale and reverse the motion. Roll your shoulders backward and down as you exhale. Relax your facial muscles and breathe slowly and deeply. Roll your shoulders ten times in each direction.

HAND-STRENGTHENING EXERCISES

You should start a hand-strengthening program only after your body is brought back into balance by regularly performing the twelve-step program detailed in Chapters 3 and 4. Your joints and muscles must be aligned and free of pain to work efficiently and be able to grow stronger. I don't believe in the old saying, "no pain, no gain." Actual pain – not the discomfort that may come from exercise – tells you that there is something wrong. If you have the patience to follow a healing program, your

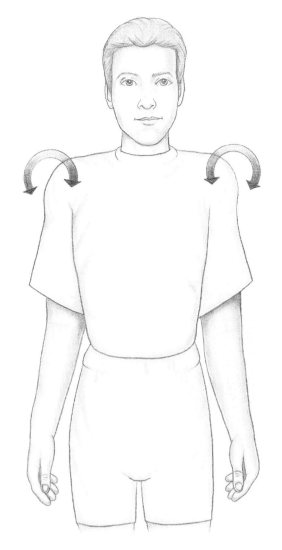

recovery time will be decreased and you can soon return to a productive, balanced life and enjoy your activities.

Remember, continual body maintenance is a must if you are to remain productive and free of muscular aches and pains. Once you are pain-free, you should regularly perform these exercises to keep balanced and help prevent future injuries or problems.

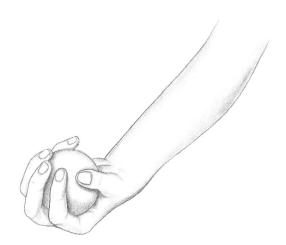

Ball squeeze for grip strength

For this exercise you need a tennis ball or a pliable rubber ball. (It's best to start with a soft, pliable bal – a Nerf ball will do – and move up to a tennis ball as you become stronger.)

Squeeze slowly and as firmly as you can without producing pain. Start with one set of ten repetitions, two to three times a day. Repeat with the other hand. Increase the number of sets as you get stronger.

Chinese ball exercise

For this, you need two Chinese exercise balls, hollow chrome balls that you can buy in most natural health stores. Rotate the balls in the palm of one hand to stimulate the energy in your fingers and hand. It will help improve circulation of vital energy throughout your body. Rotate the balls ten times, two to three times a day. Repeat with the other hand. Increase the number of rotations as you become stronger.

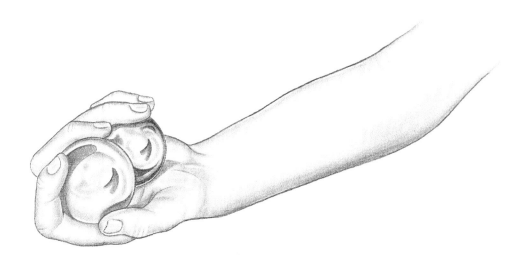

Rubber band exercise

This exercise helps increase the strength of the tendons and muscles in your hand and fingers.

Place the rubber band around your fingers, as shown. Open and close your fingers, pushing against the tension of the rubber band. Do one set of ten repetitions, two to three times a day. Repeat with your other hand. Increase the number of sets as your finger muscles become stronger. When you get stronger and this exercise becomes easy, you may want to switch to a stronger rubber band with more tension for increased resistance.

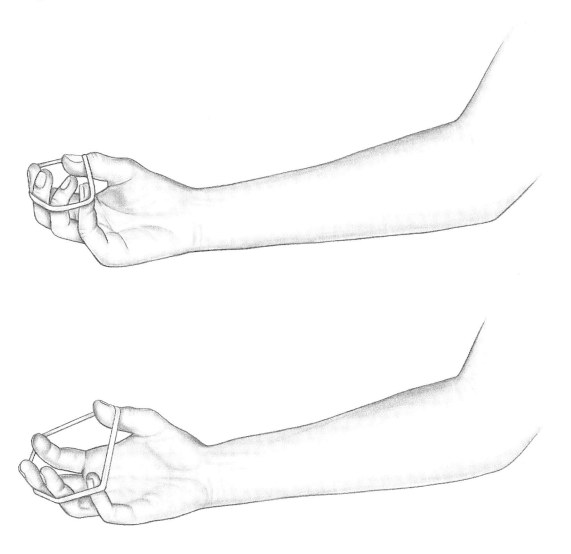

WRIST, BICEPS, AND TRICEPS EXERCISES

Do not do weight exercises until you've done the twelve-step program and your elbows and wrists are in alignment. Only when you are pain-free and healthy should you begin a strengthening routine. Trying to strengthen a misaligned joint that has tight and sore muscles will not give you the result you're seeking.

Be aware that exercise "pain" and injury pain are different – recognize the difference! Never hold your breath – the will stop the flow of energy into your muscles. Breathe evenly.

If you have never done any weight training before, it is especially important to use light weights and increase the number of repetitions gradually. If you go too fast in your training, tendinitis can develop. Start slowly and be patient! Too much too soon will slow your progress toward strong and stable joints.

For these exercises you need a one-pound weight available at sporting goods stores or a sixteen-ounce can from your pantry.

Forward wrist curls

First inhale, then exhale as you lift the weight slowly; inhale as you lower it. Start with one set of ten repetitions, two to three times a day. Breathe slowly and deeply. Repeat with your other wrist. You can increase the number of sets as you become stronger.

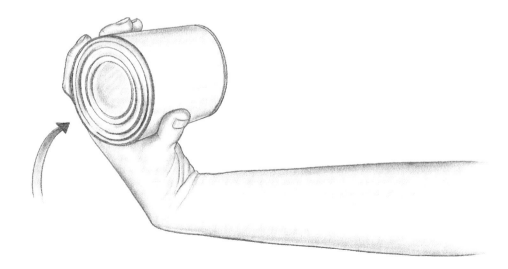

Reverse wrist curls

To do these, first flip your arm over. Inhale, then exhale as you lift the weight slowly; and inhale as you lower it. Start with one set of ten repetitions, two to three times a day. Breathe slowly and deeply. Repeat with your other wrist. You can increase the number of sets as you become stronger.

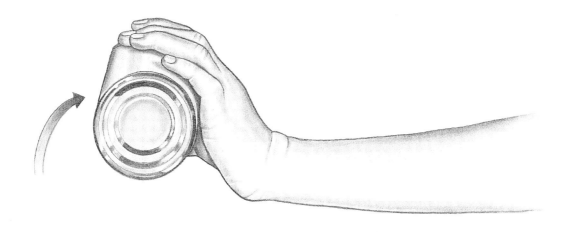

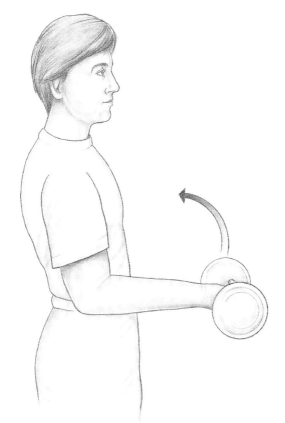

Elbow and upper arm: biceps curls

For these exercises, you need a two-pound weight, or a thirty-two-ounce can from your pantry.

Place your arm close to your side, with your elbow bent at a ninety-degree angle. Inhale, and then exhale as you slowly lift the weight; inhale as you slowly lower it. Breathe slowly and deeply. Start with on set of ten repetitions, two to three times a day. Repeat with your other arm. Increase the number of sets as you become stronger.

Elbow and upper arm triceps curls

For these exercises, you need a two-pound weight, or a thirty-two-ounce can from your pantry.

Grasping the weight, lift your arm to head level. Your elbow should be bent, with your forearm at a ninety-degree angle to your shoulder, with your opposite hand supporting your elbow, as shown. Inhale, then exhale as you slowly lift the weight toward the ceiling. Inhale as you slowly lower the weight. Breathe slowly and deeply. Repeat with your other arm. Always support your elbow joint, and start with one set of ten repetitions, two to three times a day. Increase the number of sets as you become stronger.

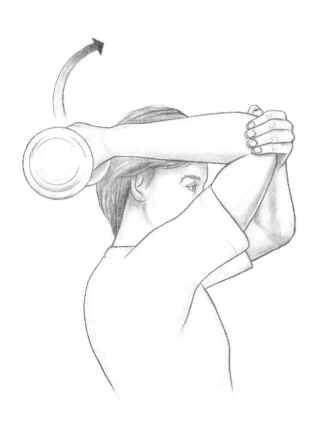
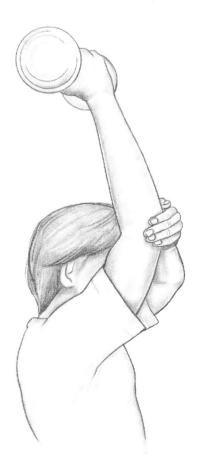

ARM AND SHOULDER STRENGTHENING EXERCISES

The aim of these four exercises is to strengthen and tone your upper arm and shoulder muscles. For these exercises, begin with a one or two-pound weight, and as you progress, gradually increase to five pounds. How soon you increase the weight depends on the health of your muscles and tendons and your overall health as well. If you have been injured, begin by doing one set of five to ten repetitions for two weeks. When you can do three sets of ten repetitions easily for a week, increase the weight by two pounds. If this feels like too much, increase it by one pound. The goal is to increase tendon strength first, and then tone the muscle as you train. This takes one to two months. Have patience – the results are long lasting!

When finished, rub the neurolymphatic reflex points for your upper arms, shoulders, neck, upper back, and chest, as shown in Chapter 5.

Lateral arm raises

Begin with one arm at a time. While standing, hold the weight in your hand at your side. Inhale, then exhale as you lift the weight straight out from your side to shoulder level. Hold for a two-second count: *one-thousand-and-one, one-thousand-and-two.* Inhale and slowly lower the weight to your side.

Do this exercise five to ten times, and then repeat with your other arm.

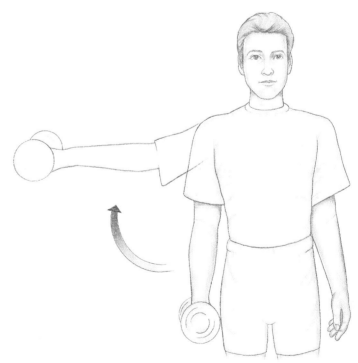

Forward arm raises

Begin with one arm at a time. While standing, hold the weight in your hand at your side, palm down. Inhale, then exhale as you lift the weight straight out in front of you to shoulder level. Hold for a two-second count: *one-thousandand-one, one-thousand-two.* Inhale and slowly lower the weight to your side. Do this exercise five to ten times. Repeat with your other arm.

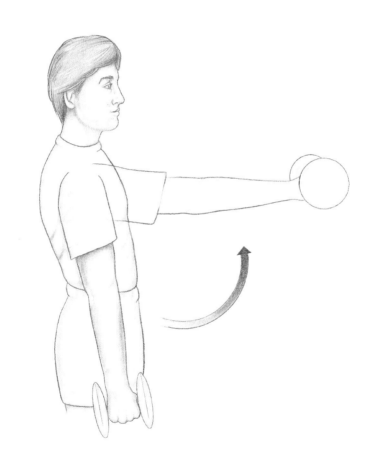

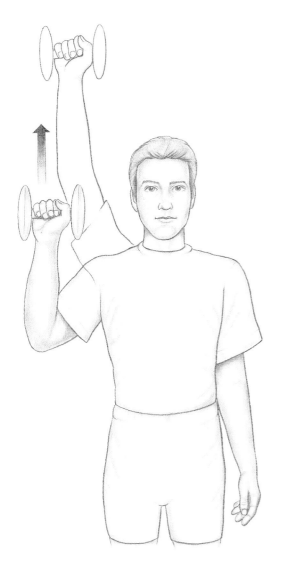

To-the-sky arm raise

Begin with one arm at a time. While standing, hold the weight in your hand; with your arm at your side, bend your elbow so the weight is roughly at shoulder level. Inhale, then exhale as you lift the weight straight above your head. Hold for a two-second count, *one-thousand-and-one, one-thousand-and-two,* then inhale as you slowly lower the weight to your side. Do this exercise five to ten times. Repeat with your other arm.

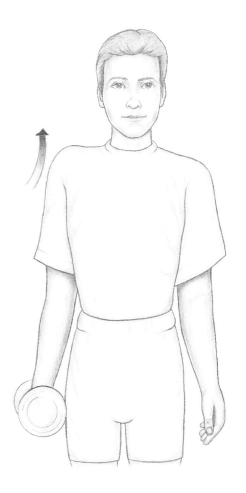

Shoulder shrugs

While standing, hold the weight in your hand at your side. Inhale, and then exhale as you raise your shoulder toward your ear. Hold for a two-second count: *one-thousand-and-one, one-thousand-and-two.* Inhale and slowly lower your shoulder. Do this exercise five to ten times. Repeat with your other arm.

Muscle Balance

Preventative stretching and strengthening of the flexor and extensor muscles of the arm and hand can help to correct the muscle strength imbalance that exists between these two muscle groups. Most ergonomic programs and exercise tools are not designed to address the actual causes of repetitive strain injuries.

Squeezing and Gripping Devices are used to exercise and strengthen the flexor muscle group. The flexor muscles are already overdeveloped from performing repetitive activities that require "closing" of the hand and using a "pinch grip" with the fingers. When you only use a gripping and squeezing device, you duplicate the exact same motion that caused the muscle imbalance in the first place. This movement when repetitive, will continue to increase the strength and rigidity of the flexor muscles exacerbating the injury even further.

Flexor and extensor muscles are opposing muscles, like front to back. In muscle balancing, there has to be balance of opposing muscle groups in order to eliminate an injury. When you begin a strengthening program, include both flexor and extensor exercises for the forearm. It is the combination of flexor and extensor movements together that corrects the muscle imbalance and can alleviate all symptoms of carpal tunnel syndrome and repetitive strain injuries.

Letters from...

P.J. Shepard

Dear Kate'... I'm glad to hear that you are still working to improve the lives of folks suffering through RSI. In 1996 when my parents were caring for me at their home in San Diego, my first outing was to a coffee shop for my stepmother to have a cup on the way to the drugstore to pick up my medication. On a high round table there was a local newspaper with a front-page article featuring you and your work. I bought your Montgomery Method book and an 8" by 11" laminated card with your exercises on it. The exercises work very well for me even though my EMG's were negative for Carpal Tunnel, I still had all the symptoms.

Now, six years later thanks to many different types of therapy and medication, still ongoing though, but much less frequently, I work full time and have a life again. Thank you for the part you have played and continue to play in my recovery. I have your "At A Glance" card of the twelve steps on my wall at work, mostly to show others, as I can do the exercises blindfolded now.

Acting chairperson EBRSI
Newsletter posted by the ctdrn.org site (Cumulative Trauma Disorder Resource Network)

Wrist Braces and Splints

Wrist Braces and Splints: Wrist braces and splints are not effective in hand and wrist injuries, i.e. carpal tunnel syndrome (CTS) and other repetitive strain injuries (RSI). The idea behind these devices is to keep the wrist from dropping into flexion so that the wrist stays in a neutral position in order to reduce impingement of the median nerve going through the carpal tunnel. Instead, wrist braces often increase the symptoms because of the abnormal inactivity of the muscles that decreases circulation and sense of awareness.

Wrist braces are NOT GOOD to wear while performing daily activities because they tell your extensor muscles that hold your hand up, they don't have to work anymore. Over time the muscles can atrophy from nonuse and become weak. The wrist brace works as a "crutch," eliminating muscle movement. The imbalance between the flexors and extensor then becomes even greater.

Another major problem while wearing a wrist brace is even though the wrist is still in a neutral position, you can still use your fingers to perform repetitive or static flexion movements, such as typing and writing. This will increase more stress on the tendons and muscles of the fingers, and continued imbalance develops.

Refer to the resource section in the back of the book for a list of devices that are available for balancing the flexor and extensor muscles. This is a limited list but may be of help to you.

Warm-Up Stretches for Your Hands

Just as you should warm-up and stretch before you begin an athletic activity such as running or playing softball, you should warm-up and stretch your hands before they begin their day of activity. Begin each day with these warm-up exercises. They are designed to increase your range of motion and the glide of your tendons, and to stretch the muscles of your hands and fingers. They can be done any time and any place. Remember to breathe slowly and deeply with each exercise to maintain the energy flow throughout your body.

Hand Circles. Gently rotate each wrist in loose circles, five times clockwise, and five times counterclockwise.

Fist Clinches. Open and close your fists rapidly five times.

Wrist Bends. Stretch on wrist forward and backward, using the opposite hand to gently push the wrist into a stretch. Hold for a four-second count in each direction. Repeat with your other wrist.

Finger Bends. Stretch your fingers forward and backward, one at a time, using your other hand to gently push. Hold for a count of one or two seconds. Repeat with your other hand.

Finger Rotations. Gently grasp the fingers of the opposite hand. Rotate each finger clockwise, and then counterclockwise, one at a time. Use the opposite hand to help do the exercise, then repeat with your other hand.

Finger Pulls. Pull gently on you fingers, grasping the finger joint closest to the palm. Repeat with your other hand.

Hand Shakes. Holding your arms loosely at your sides, shake your hands gently, one at a time.

Finger Spread. Spread your fingers wide apart and stretch your fingers outward. Repeat.

Finger-Palm Touch. One at a time, touch the pad of each finger and your thumb to the palm of your hand. You should be able to touch your pads to the palm of your hand easily. Repeat on the other hand.

Finger-Joint Bend. Holding the tip of each finger, individually bend each joint of that finger. Do not force a joint to bend. Work gradually with the joint to increase flexibility.

Finger Pinch. Pinch the ends of each finger firmly but gently for a one-second count. This stimulates energy in the six meridians in the Chinese acupuncture system. Repeat on the other hand.

Palm Rub. Rub the palms of your hands together rapidly for a friction rub. Then gently massage your hands and fingers. This is a good way to increase circulation.

Chapter 7

Ergonomics: How to Work Pain Free

Ergonomics is the applied science that seeks to fit your job to you through evaluation and design of the work environment in relation to human characteristics and interactions in the workplace. This includes the type of equipment used; chair, desk, and monitor heights; arm and wrist rests as needed; footstool, and so on. It also includes ensuring that everything is adjusted to fit your body comfortably so you can work safely.

SETTING UP THE WORK STATION

Whenever you arrive for work or sit down at your home computer – or your Nintendo or Sega play station – you should take five minutes to adjust the station. The time you take can save you from an uncomfortable workday and much wear and tear on your body. All your equipment should be adjusted to fit your body comfortably – taking into account your height and size – so you can function comfortably for the entire workday. The dimensions of the workstation layout will vary depending on your height, arm reach, leg length, and general size.

You need to consider five factors in setting up your work station:

- whether the equipment supports your body comfortably
- layout of the work station
- size of the area
- adjustability for each person
- whether the environment is enjoyable or pleasant to work in

Correct work station preparation is especially important for mental concentration and physical relaxation to maximize work efficiency and productivity. Developing the habit of correct preparation at the work station can save hours of inefficient and unproductive time because of musculoskeletal discomfort and pain.

Remember your environment! A lack of fresh air, which is common in many offices with sealed windows, poor lighting, and too much noise all make your workday more difficult. You can't do much about windows that do not open, but adding a few plants to your office can help purify the air. Fluorescent lights or lights in the wrong position can add to eye strain or cause headaches in some people. Use a lamp with a regular light bulb instead of an overhead fluorescent light. Try to minimize noise. Wear soft foam earplugs if you cannot decrease the noise around you.

All About Your Chair

Your chair protects the curvature of your spine. It should support the low, middle, and upper curve of your spine to prevent slouching. This reduces strain on your neck, shoulders, back, arms, hands, hips, legs, and feet. Optimal heights for a chair and desk or workbench depend on your proportions. Your chair should be at a height that allows your feet to be flat on the floor. It should have safe and easy-to-use control knobs.

There are many kinds of chairs suitable for work. If you are buying one, take your time shopping. Sit in different models. Choose the one that best fits your body. Remember, you will spend many hours in this chair. It should accommodate your needs. Here are some things to look for (also see illustration that follows this section):

Seat. The seat itself should fit you correctly. It should not be so deep that you cannot use the back rest or so long that it puts pressure on the back of your knees or calves, which could inhibit circulation. It should have a rounded front edge, which will minimize pressure on the back of your thighs. The fabric should be non-slip and of a breathable material, with enough padding to give comfort. Chairs with wheels or casters are best, as they decrease fatigue from having to get up and down – you can just roll instead of getting up or reaching too far. The wheels should not restrict movement, and the chair should be designed to protect against tipping over or falling.

Back rest. The backrest should fit the contour of your back to maintain the natural curvature of your spine. It should give firm support for your lower and middle back, with enough padding for comfort. There should be an adjustable knob for the lower back. If not, put a medium to firm pillow in the curve of your low back, which will help eliminate back fatigue.

Arm rest. Armrests are recommended for all types of chairs, unless they get in the way of the work. They should be padded and wide enough for elbow comfort, but not so wide that you cannot use them. The height and distance apart should provide comfortable support that allows for easy movement and correct positioning of your chair.

Once you have a good chair, adjusting it is crucial. You'll need to adjust the seat, the armrests, backrest, and footrest. Your chair seat should incline slightly forward to transfer pressure from your spine to your thighs and feet. If you use different chairs throughout the day, take the time to adjust the chair to fit you. It can mean many more hours of productive and comfortable work.

A few tips to remember:

- Adjust the seat to proper working height, so that your feet can sit flat on the floor and your knees are approximately two to four inches below the top of the desk
- Adjust the lumbar curve (the part that fits into and above the small of your back) to protect the curve of your lower back. If you do not have an adjustable lumbar knob, put a small pillow in the curve of your lower back for support.

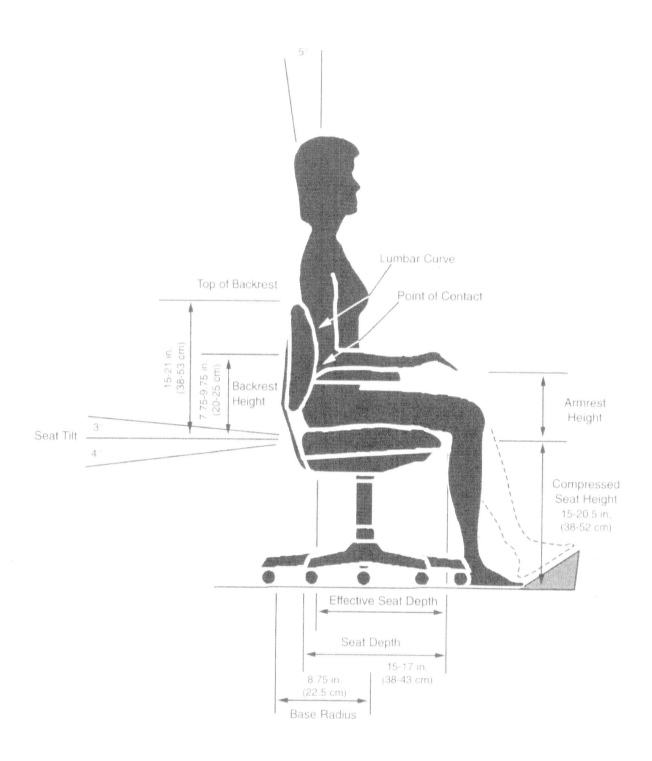

Other Work Station Details

Footrest. A footrest will help take the strain off your upper legs, which allows better circulation through your knees and lower legs. It should have complete contact with the floor and have a base of at least twenty-six inches. It should not be able to roll; if it has wheels or casters, they should be of the locking type. Footrests are used to help bring your upper legs parallel to the floor.

Computer monitor. The top of the screen should be at eye level, with your eyes cast down slightly, as shown on page 105, to see the center of the screen. Adjust your computer monitor to a height that allows you to do this comfortably. Lowering the screen may help achieve a more suitable viewing angle and alleviate the strain on your eye muscles.

Desk height. The height of your desk or workstation should be at waist level, which is determined by the height of your chair. A work area that is too high will create stressful shoulder and arm positions. An area that is too low will cause stressful bending of the neck and trunk of the body.

Keyboard angle. The surface of the desk on which the keyboard rests should be arranged to keep your wrist in a neutral position. It's best to use a three-fourth-inch pad or wrist rest in front of your keyboard, which you can find at any office or computer supply store. You should not, however, use the support to rest your wrists on. Instead, use it to help keep your wrists in a neutral position, suspended in a straight position rather than bent. Do not lean on it this will increase pressure on the median nerve. Also, if you use the small collapsible legs on the back of your keyboard, make sure you use a wrist pad to prevent an awkward position of your hands. If your keyboard is sitting on top of a standard desk, you may want to request or buy a keyboard tray that fits under the desk. A lower keyboard will often allow for less tension on the muscles of your forearm and your elbow and wrist joints.

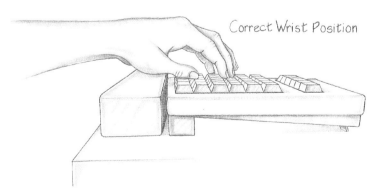
Correct Wrist Position

Mouse. If you use a mouse frequently, make sure it fits your hand comfortably. The mouse should support your whole palm, and you should not have to grasp it with your fingers. Your wrist should stay in a neutral, not flexed, position. All the muscles of your fingers and hand should be relaxed, using very little pressure to push the clicker button. All hands are not the same size! To find a comfortable mouse, e-mail Contour Design at info@contour-design.com. They have designed a mouse with five different right and left hand sizes – extra small, small, medium, large, and extra large. Contact the Web site at www.contourdesign.com or call 800-462-6678. If you spend a lot of time using your mouse, you may want to decrease mouse time by learning keyboard shortcut commands for specific things you frequently use the mouse for. For instance, you can close many word processing programs by hitting the control key and *S* key, rather than using the mouse.

Document holder. Use a document holder, available at office supply stores, to hold paperwork so you can keep your head upright while typing. Looking down can continually irritate your cervical vertebrae and damage your nerves and spinal disks, thereby contributing to muscle weakness.

Phone headset. If you need to continue working or to have both hands free while talking on the phone, request or invest in a headset for your phone, or use a speaker-phone. This prevents you from straining your neck and shoulder muscles and getting your body out of alignment while hunching one shoulder up to hold the phone to your ear.

WORK STATION DESIGN

A well-designed workstation can cut down on the number of times you must reach too far with your arms. On the following page is an example an efficient workstation.

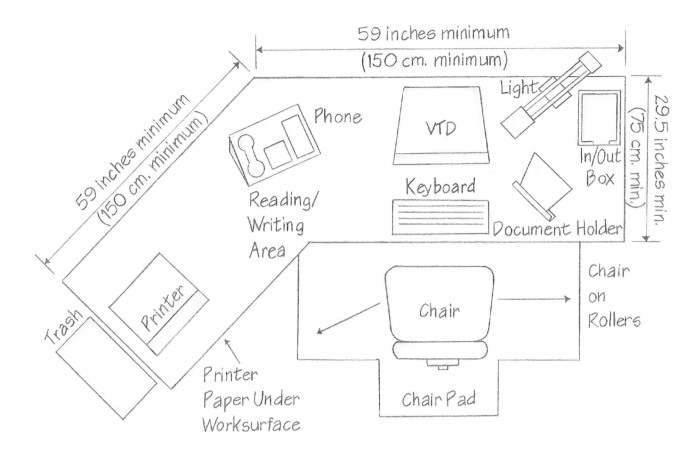

The work station should allow you to face forward. You should be able to reach the items you use often with a normal reach without stretching, straining, or twisting. Having a chair with coasters and a hard surface to slide on will help cut down on overreach situations.

- Avoid reaching behind you and twisting your spine backward
- Avoid reaching across your body with one or two hands and twisting forward
- Avoid overreaching by putting items within arms' length
- Limit frequent, fast, and forceful movements
- Be sure there are no obstructions in the work area.

Protect Your Wrists

At any routine activity, you want to avoid putting your hands in compromising positions that can aggravate your arms and wrist joints. For example, if you use a keyboard all day with your wrists in the wrong position, you can feel numbness and tingling because of hyperextension of your wrist joint. Take a look at the illustrations below to see correct and incorrect positions.

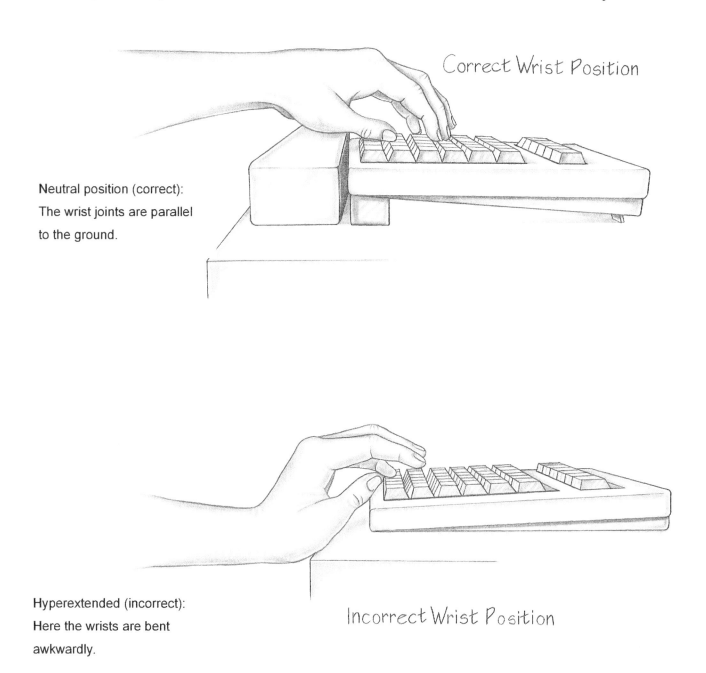

Correct Wrist Position

Neutral position (correct):
The wrist joints are parallel
to the ground.

Hyperextended (incorrect):
Here the wrists are bent
awkwardly.

Incorrect Wrist Position

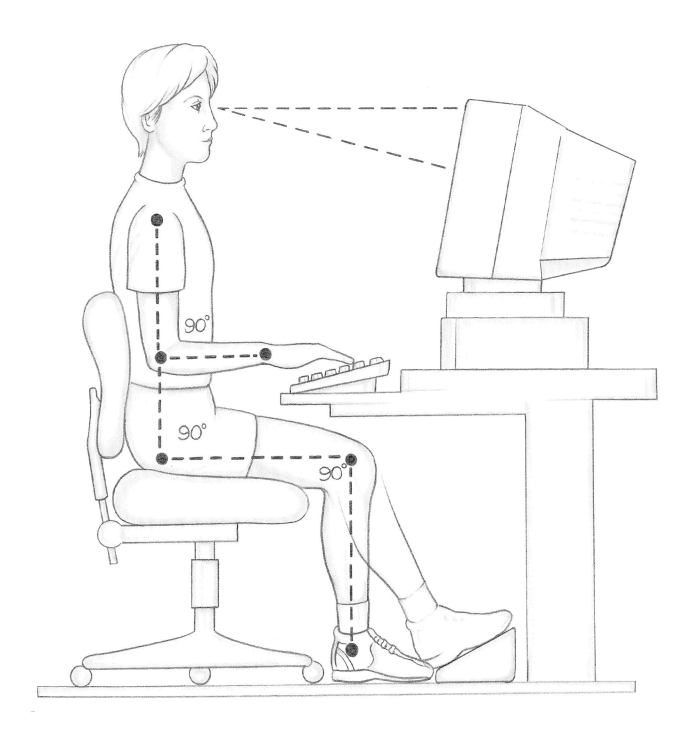

THE IMPORTANCE OF GOOD POSTURE

Correct posture allows for increased blood flow throughout the body and reduces harmful compression of the spine. Good posture at a work station starts with sitting up straight with proper support along the curve of your spine. Here are the basic guidelines of good posture:

- Your back tilts slightly backward to increase the distance between your torso and thighs, and your thighs are at a ninety-degree angle to your torso

- Your shoulders are down and slightly backward, free of stress

- Your arms are relaxed

- Your forearms are at ninety-degree angles to the floor

- Your wrists and hands are in a neutral position, supported and slightly elevated – not resting on the desk or a wrist pad

- Your feet are flat on the floor or on a footrest

- Your head is erect with your eyes directed slightly down to view the computer screen.

Letters from...

A Legal Assistant

At the time I met Kate' Montgomery, I was a part time student and full time legal assistant. I began having numbness and pain in my wrists and hands. One of my friends referred me to Kate's book. Kate' lived in San Diego and since I lived in San Diego too, I tracked her down. I booked an appointment with her. When I spoke with Kate', the first thing she said was "don't do the surgery, carpal tunnel can be reversed". At first, I was a little skeptical, after all I had gone to many doctors and they all had recommended the same, "surgery."

In my desperate state and trying to find a solution, I decided to put myself in her hands. I followed everything she said in her book. After a few sessions with her and doing the exercises, my hands began to recover their strength and I was beginning to perform normal things like cooking, lifting heavy objects, and using my computer again without much pain. I did not have to quit my job and regained all hopes of recovering without surgery. It has been two years since that faithful day, and my hands have recovered fully. Thanks Kate' for being that wonderful medicine woman you are!!!!

_ Yinia Najar

WHY YOU MUST TAKE REST BREAKS

In today's workplace, correct postural alignment of the body is necessary to avoid the physical aches and pains that come from using improper equipment or equipment that is inadequate to support your physical structure. Businesses spend thousands of dollars a year on ergonomically safe office equipment to ensure the comfort of each employee. But even if you have ergonomically safe and well-designed equipment in your work space, you may have the same physical aches and pains as you did before – if you don't take adequate rest breaks.

Besides using your equipment safely, you must remember to stretch throughout the day and take frequent rest breaks. In an eight-hour workday you need cycles of work and rest to stay pro-ductive and healthy. To avoid strain and tension in your muscles, it's necessary to stop and take several rest breaks throughout the day.

> *Work Station Check List*
>
> **At your seat:**
>
> - Is your back tilted slightly backward?
> - Are your thighs at right angles to your torso?
> - Are your shoulders down and slightly backward?
> - Are your arms relaxed?
> - Are your forearms at right angles to the floor?
> - Are your wrists and hands in a neutral position, not resting on anything?
> - Are your feet flat on the floor or a footrest?
> - Is your head erect, with your line of vision slightly down?
> - Is your back rest set to fit the contour of your back?
> - Is your computer monitor set so you look slightly down at it rather than up?
> - Is your desk or work station at waist level?
> - Are your wrists level while you use your keyboard?
> - Is your workspace arranged so you can reach things easily?

Even if you are rushed, it's crucial to pause in your work periodically. You don't save time by skipping breaks: The fatigue you feel will affect your productivity. Without breaks you increase the risk of musculoskeletal injury.

Each person is unique, and the risk of injury varies with how much continuous and repetitive work you are doing. Some may need longer periods of rest to recover. Spend your rest breaks correcting posture and doing techniques to help align and stretch your body. (These are summarized in Chapter 8.) Use your lunch period to prepare your body to work the second half of the day, by running through the twelve steps of the carpal tunnel ritual. (If you don't have time to do all of them, concentrate on steps one through eleven.)

Letters from...

A Longtime Computer User

Your book has been a miracle resource for me in dealing with pain in my arms and wrists for 10+ years of mouse use. I reviewed 7 or 8 books on RSI and Carpal Tunnel. The techniques in this book include actions that are "manageable" and require 15-20 minutes. Other books were suggesting a complete life makeover! I used these techniques and my pain was 75% gone... I hope to have a full recovery soon. I don't have health insurance and thanks to your book I have been able to rehabilitate myself. So a very special thanks for this book."

– Gavin Khan

HOW TO PROTECT YOUR EYES

Creating a safe working environment protects the body from possible risks-including those to your eyes. Adjusting your work station is essential to avoid eye strain. Correct posture and support are necessary to allow your eyes to focus correctly. Your eyes naturally lower to forty degrees from the horizontal line of sight. This is a coordinated movement that works in conjunction with focusing and other eye movements. If you use a computer, make sure the screen is at the correct height to avoid muscle strain in your eyes. The screen should be lowered for a better viewing angle, slightly below the horizon.

Here are some things you can do to help reduce stress while sitting at a computer monitor:

- Make sure your chair height and monitor height fit your body's measurements and that your body is totally supported and comfortable
- Increases oxygen flow to our brain, relaxes our muscles, and helps us focus more easily

- Take breaks. Getting up, moving around, and stretching increase circulation in our muscles and release tension in our body. Breaks are important to ensure a more productive and efficient workday.

RELAXATION TECHNIQUES FOR YOUR EYES

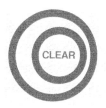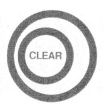

This exercise is to be done before you start work, as many times a day as you can, and at the end of the day. Eye muscles need downtime because as long as your eyes are open, these muscles are working. You especially need to do this exercise if you are going to be involved in intense, close work or staring at a computer monitor several hours a day.

Relaxation palming. While seated at your desk, place your elbows on a cushion, shoulder-width apart. Close your eyes. Put your hands over your eyes, covering your eyes but not applying any pressure. Now relax and breathe deeply. With each breath, relax your facial muscles and feel the tension leave. If you see flashes of light or shadows, ignore them until the darkness returns. Continue to breathe even more deeply. Feel the tension draining from your eyes, face, and body.

Palm-friction rub. You can get an extra enhancement by rubbing your palms vigorously together, to create heat and energy in your hands. Place your hands lightly over your eyes, letting the warmth of your hands penetrate your eye muscles. Continue to breathe deeply and evenly throughout this exercise. Do this as often as needed throughout the day.

Convergence relaxation. Convergence is the aiming of the eyes toward each other as you look at objects nearby. Your eyes can be overworked when you are doing excessive amounts of close work. The following technique is designed to help you relax your eyes when they are converging for long periods.

First, focus your eyes on a blank wall at least ten feet away from you. Move this page, with the circles, slowly into your line of sight at your normal reading distance. Keep your eyes focused on the wall, however.

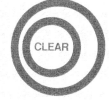

You should begin to see three, rather than two, sets of circles. If you see four sets of circles, try to bring the middle two sets together by concentrating. Of the three sets, the one in the middle – the one that's not really there – should appear as a three-dimensional figure. The smaller circle should appear closer to you than the larger circle. If this is difficult to visualize, try moving the circles slowly toward yourself while you focus on the wall. This can be difficult to do at first, but this is a very effective procedure, so keep trying. Once you have seen the central ring as three-dimensional, try to bring the word *clear* into focus. This will ensure that your eyes are focused properly as well as turned in the right direction. Do this technique for about ten minutes a day, preferably in the earlier part of the day and before doing intense, close work.

Convergence stimulation. If your eyes have difficulty converging, then you may experience tiring, general fatigue, or double vision while doing near work. This technique is designed to enhance your ability to converge your eyes so they can align their respective images properly. It is the opposite of the convergence relaxation technique.

Hold this page at your normal reading distance. You should see two sets of concentric circles. This time put the tip of a pencil midway between the circles and focus on it. Keep looking at the tip of the pencil during the entire procedure. Move the pencil slowly toward your eyes, leaving the illustration in place. Be aware of the circles beyond the end of the pencil as you do so.

When the pencil is about six inches from your eyes, you should begin to see three, rather than two, sets of concentric circles. The set in the middle – the one that isn't really there – should appear as a three-dimensional figure, with the smaller circle seeming farther away from you than the larger one. Keep the pencil still, and keep looking at it. Your eyes should feel as if they are crossing. Now try to bring the word *clear* into focus while maintaining the three-dimensional effect. Once you have done this, look away from the circles. Then try the exercise again. Do this exercise until it becomes easy to see and maintain the three-dimensional effect and the image is clear. As with the previous exercise, move the circles in and out once you can easily maintain the effect. These exercises should be done at least twice a day. Eye health is an important factor to consider when using a computer for long periods of time. Children especially need to do these exercises to prevent unnecessary eyestrain and possible early eye damage. For more information on Dr. Anshel and his vision program, refer to the resource section.

Chapter 8

The Montgomery Method: A Daily Maintenance Plan

SELF ASSESSMENT STEPS (1-7)

Step 1: Tinel's Test

Step 2: *Phalen's Test*

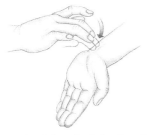

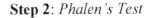
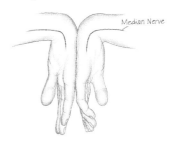

Step 3: *Muscle Monitoring*

Step 4: *Perceived Grip Strength*

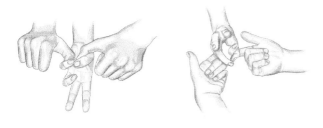

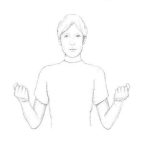

Step 5: *Fingerpad Sensitivity*

Step 6: *Palpation of the Muscles*

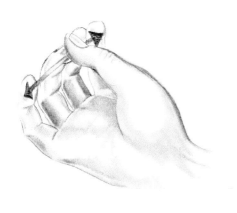

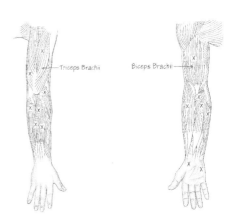

Step 7: *Pain Level: 1-10, 10 the most pain, rate your pain level.*

THE MONTGOMERY METHOD (1 – 6)

Step 1: *Posture correction*

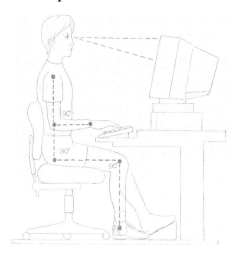

Step 2: *Neck Massage*

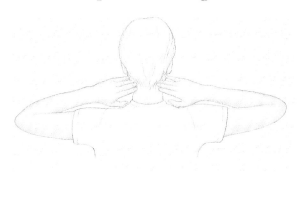

Step 3: *Shoulder Rolls*

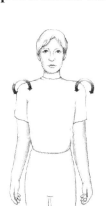

Step 4: *Forward arm extension*

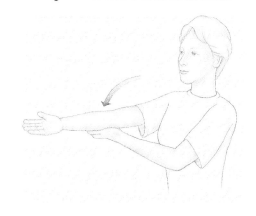

Step 5: *Lateral arm extension*

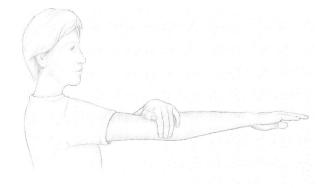

Step 6: *Wrist press*

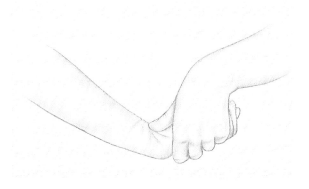

THE MONTGOMERY METHOD (7 – 11)

Step 7: *Wrist Pull*   **Step 8**: *Wrist squeeze*

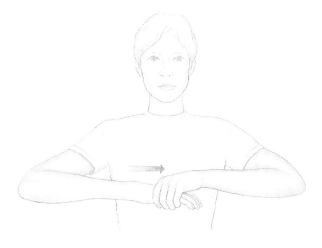   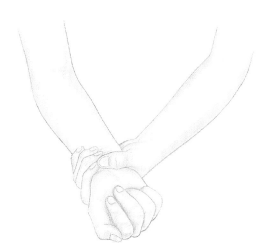

Step 9: *Finger pull*   **Step 10**: *Upper back stretch*

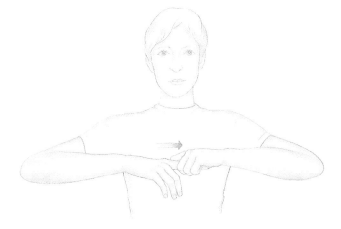

Step 11: *Shoulder, chest, and elbow stretch*

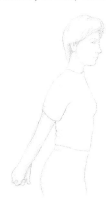

Step 12: *Muscle Therapy*

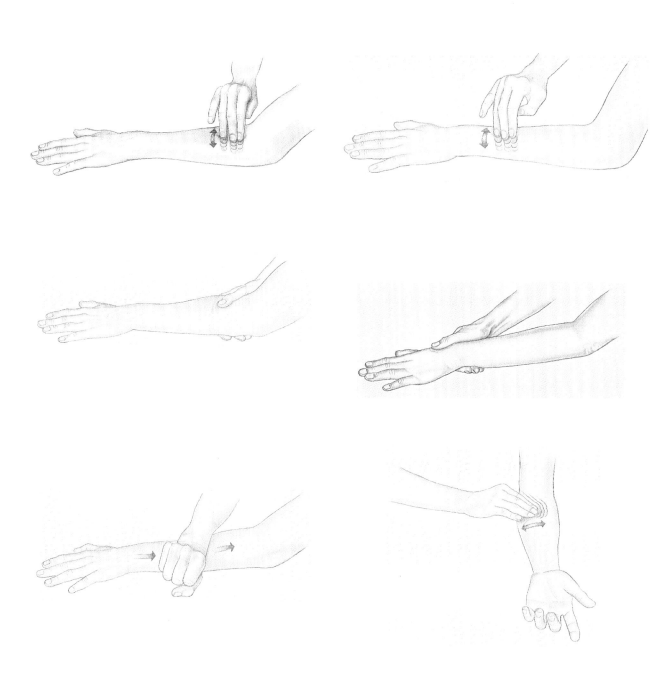

Step 12: *Muscle Therapy*

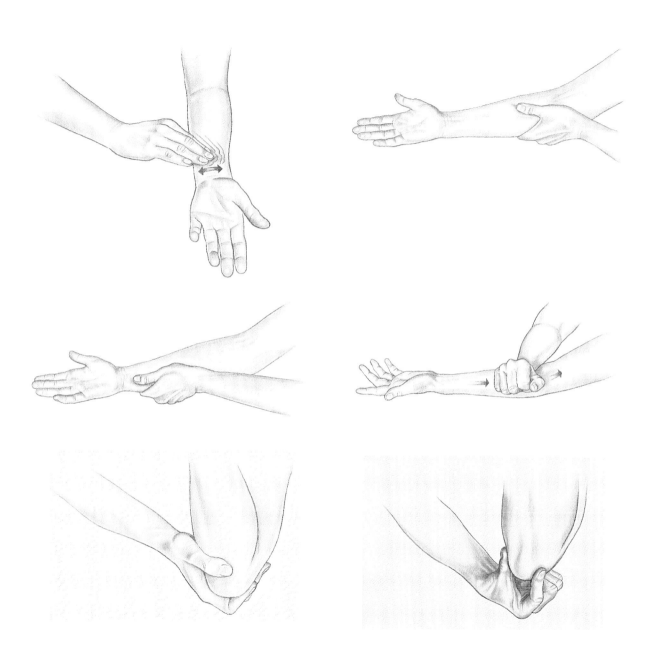

Step 12: *Muscle Therapy*

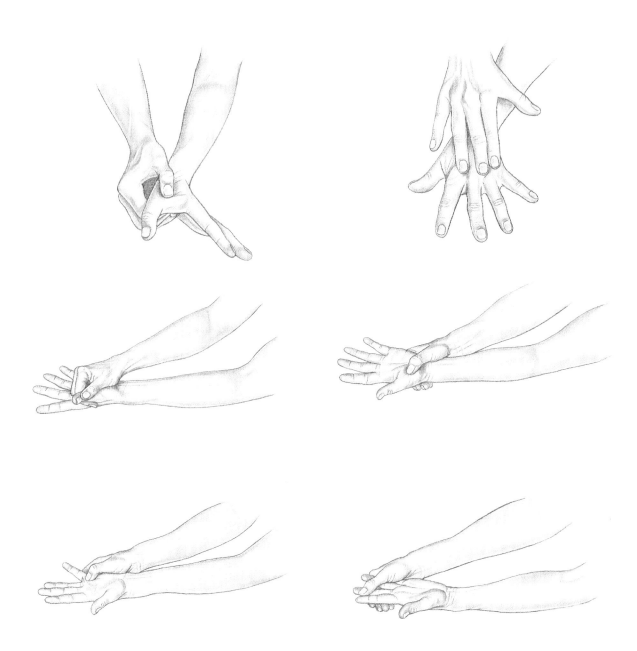

THE MYOFACIAL STRETCH AND RELEASE TECHNIQUE
Extensor Forearm Muscles

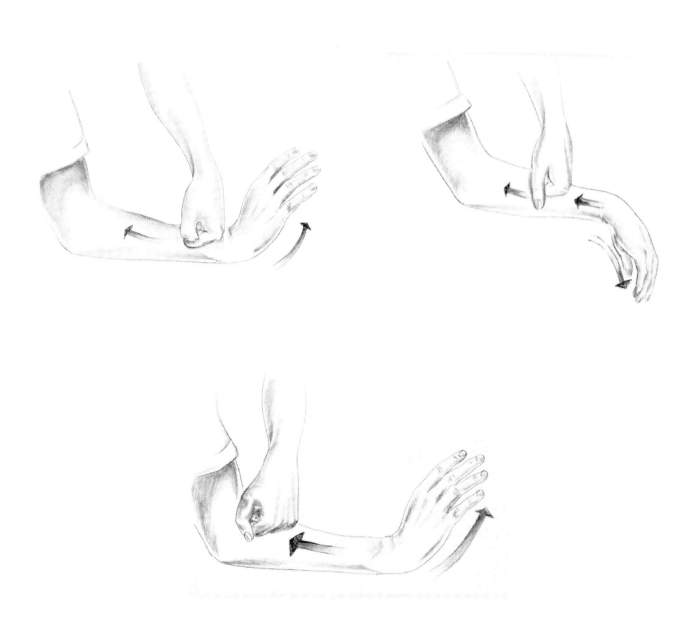

THE MYOFACIAL STRETCH AND RELEASE TECHNIQUE
Flexor Forearm Muscles

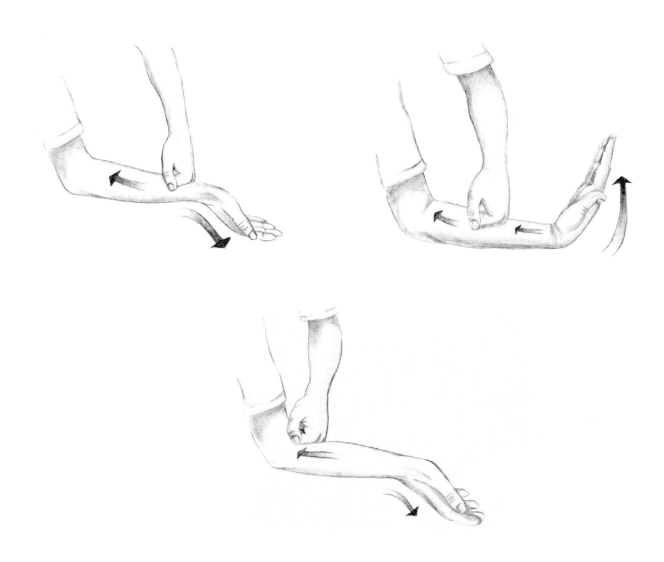

STRETCHING PROGRAM

Checking range of motion

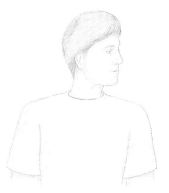

Neck release

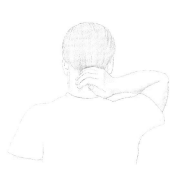

Isometric stretch

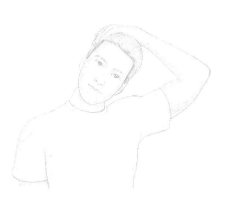

Shoulder half-circles

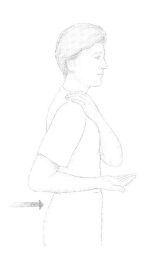

Shoulder raises full-circles

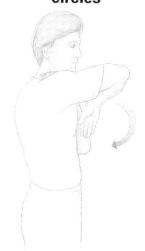

Shoulder shakes

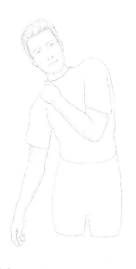

Shoulder shrugs

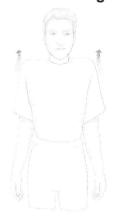

Shoulder rolls

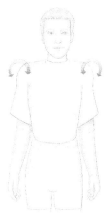

MUSCLE-STRENGTHENING EXERCISES

Ball squeeze for grip strength

Chinese ball exercise

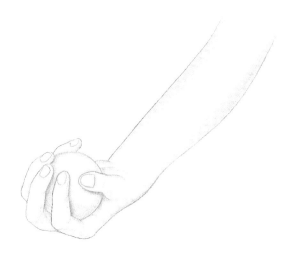

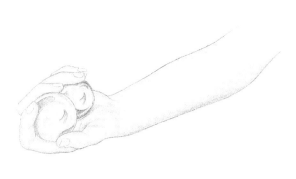

Rubber band exercise

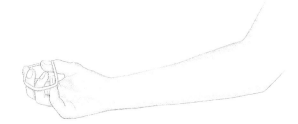

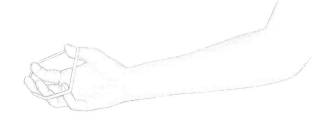

Wrist exercises

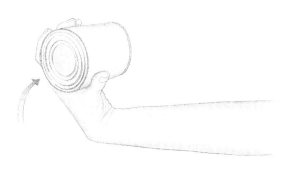

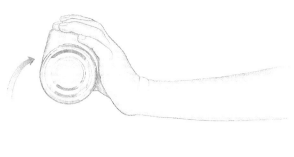

MUSCLE-STREGTHENING EXERCISES

Elbow and Upper Arm

Biceps curls

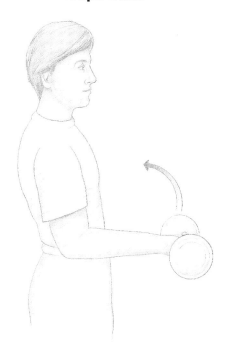

Triceps curls

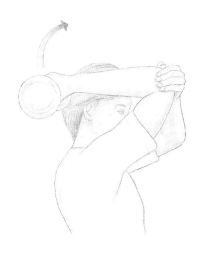

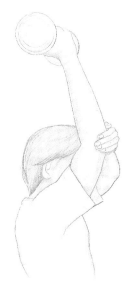

MUSCLE-STRENGTHENING EXERCISES

Arms and Shoulders

Lateral arm raises

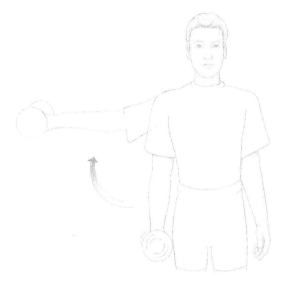

Forward arm raises

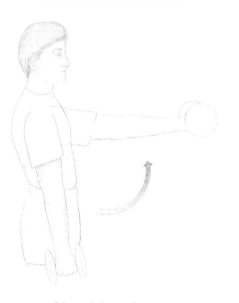

To-the-sky raises

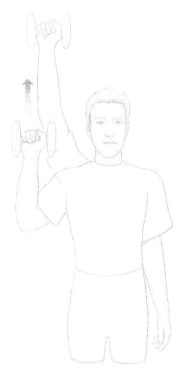

Shoulder shrugs

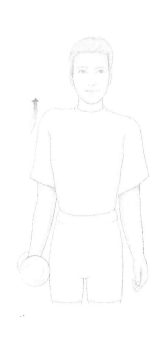

HAND WARM-UP AND STRETCHES

Once you've done the corrective measures, have achieved proper alignment, and are pain free, run these warm-ups before you begin your workday:

1. **Hand circles**
2. **Fist clinches**
3. **Wrist bends**
4. **Finger bends**
5. **Finger rotations**
6. **Finger pulls**
7. **Hand shakes**
8. **Finger spread**
9. **Finger-palm touch**
10. **Finger-thumb touch**
11. **Finger-joint bends**
12. **Finger pinch**
13. **Palm rub**

Letters from...

A Computer Instructor and Massage Therapist

I am a computer software instructor, power user of computers, and a licensed massage therapist. I have experienced the pain of carpal tunnel syndrome, particularly after a bicycle accident in which I broke both my arms. As a massage therapist, self-care is very important to my longevity in the field. I have personally used the information and techniques in Kate's book, as self-care program for my wrists and arms with great success, and I refer my students to her book as an excellent tool for the prevention and treatment of carpal tunnel syndrome.

– MIA TURPEL

WHEN YOU ARRIVE AT WORK

Because you'll likely have more time at home, you may want to run through the entire twelve-step program before leaving for work. Once you arrive, here's the routine you should follow before you begin work. Remember to breathe deeply throughout your routine and to pay attention to your breathing throughout the day, as well. Also, it's important to drink plenty of water throughout the day so you stay well hydrated.

- Make sure the equipment at your work station is comfortable, fits your body, and is placed conveniently to reduce overreaching and twisting of your body
- Whether sitting or standing, align your body. Lightly and quickly massage your neck, shoulders, and arms
- Do some neck and shoulder range-of-motion stretches. Go through the first eleven steps of the twelve-step program, especially the upper back, shoulder, chest, and elbow stretches, steps 10 and 11
- Do some general stretching, such as reaching for the sky. Total body stretching before work prepares your body for the tasks at hand. (Remember also to get out of your chair at break time to stretch.)
- Rub your neurolymphatic reflex points
- Breathing equals Energy - Remember to breathe as this keeps the your body energized. (Refer to Chapter 5)
- Water – Drink plenty of good spring water to re hydrate the body and improve mental clarity.

Break-Time Routine

For optimum performance, do these things during your break time or once every one or two hours, if possible. Remember to drink plenty of water throughout the day to avoid dehydration and to breathe deeply during the routine. Stretch and rub your reflex points as needed.

- Check your posture: Whether sitting or standing, align your body
- Massage your neck, shoulders, and arms lightly
- Do some neck and shoulder range-of-motion stretches

- Complete as much of the twelve-step method as you have time for, concentrating on the elbow and wrist exercises, steps 4-8, and the upper back, shoulder, chest, and elbow stretches, steps 10-11

- Get out of your chair and do some general stretching. Take 10 minutes out of every hour to walk away form the computer, perform stretches and range of motion exercises plus you may want to massage your arms and hands to avoid sore muscles (Chapters 4 and 6)

- This is a good time to drink a large glass of water. Staying hydrated helps keep your muscles relaxed and healthy.

After You Get Home

When you arrive home, run through the following routines. (Remember to drink plenty of spring water.)

- Check your posture
- Massage your neck, shoulder, and arms lightly
- Do neck and shoulder range-of-motion stretches
- Do the twelve-step method
- Stretch out
- Rub your neurolymphatic reflex points.

Afterward, take a hot Epsom salts bath: Add two to three cups of Epsom salts to a warm bath and soak for fifteen to twenty minutes. Relax! You will feel great in the morning. You may want to add a few drops of lavender essence, available at natural health stores, to the bath, to help soothe and calm your nervous system.

Tips for A...

Computer programmer. Before you begin your day, adjust your workstation. This takes five minutes. Every two hours you should do steps 1-11. Massage your muscles as needed. Get up and move around and stretch. Drink plenty of water. Relax your eyes with the vision relaxation exercises described in Chapter 7.

Musician. Warm-up with exercises and self-massage your arms and hands before practice or performing. Complete steps 1-11 before and after playing. Warm-up with the following exercises:

- Ball squeeze or grip strength, ten to twenty times, each hand
- Chinese ball exercise, ten times, each hand
- Rubber band exercise, ten to twenty times, each hand. Use exercise tools to stretch andstrengthen the extensor muscles as well as the flexor muscles (pinch grip) of the forearm.

Golfer. Complete steps 1-11 before you tee off. Steps 4-11 can be done throughout the game as needed. After the game, repeat all steps. Use exercise tools to stretch and strengthen the extensor muscles as well as the flexor muscles (pinch grip) of the forearm. A massage is recommended after a tournament, but never get one the day before a tournament, as it may make your body feel sluggish and toxic.

Tennis player. Complete steps 1-11 before you begin a match. Steps 4-11 can be done throughout the game as needed. After the game, repeat all steps. A massage is recommended after a tournament, but never before a tournament, as it may make your body feel sluggish and toxic. Rub the neurolymphatic reflex points for the hamstrings and quadriceps as well as the upper body. For hamstrings, rub the inside of the legs. For quadriceps, rub under the rib cage diagonally. Rub firmly for ten to thirty seconds.

***Once you have brought the body back into structural balance, incorporate stretching and strengthening exercises for the flexor and extenor muscles of the forearm.

Knitter, Needlepoint, Quilter. Be aware of your posture the whole time you are knitting, needlepointing, or quilting. Doing similar tasks. Rounded shoulders are a hazard with these hobbies. Complete steps 1-11, and stretch throughout your day. Include steps 10 and 11 as much as possible. (For more on how to use the neurolymphatic reflex points, refer to Chapter 4.)

NUTRITION AND REPETITIVE STRAIN INJURY (RSI)

Recently, a client of mine injured her wrist from a bike accident. She had the normal soreness and swelling but after a week, another week, and then a month went by and her wrist still would not heal. She went to a doctor and had it examined… no broken bones and it appeared there were no torn ligaments or tendons. Her symptoms were those of carpal tunnel and DeQuervain's syndromes. She saw a chiropractor and an acupuncturist, which seem to help temporarily, but the swelling and pain persisted. I suggested that there might be a nutritional or biochemical reason for her not being able to heal. So she did a hair analysis to see what "trend or direction" her body had taken. What possible mineral imbalances might exist?

When the results came back, the four-macro minerals (calcium, magnesium, sodium, and potassium, along with zinc and copper) that help to regulate our metabolism, thyroid and adrenal function, and oxidation rate, were out of balance. Including other minerals that are necessary to keep your body in running order. There were also toxic metals present that could be contributing to this physiological dysfunction. One major contributing factor, which I find in most of my clients, is she was also under a lot of stress and had been for a very long time.

STRESS, whether internal or external, is the most significant cause for biochemical changes in the body.

She agreed, once understanding this possible cause of her persistent swelling, to follow the recommended supplemental regimen for three months and to follow the recommended nutritional program and some additional life-style changes. To her surprise and delight, within two weeks, the pain, swelling and soreness had all but disappeared.

I began to think this was something to mention in this new edition. When the symptoms of RSI won't go away, and your other forms of therapy haven't been working as well as they could, and you may be considering surgery, you might want to consider hair analysis. It can assess the biochemical and nutritional status and help to give you more insight into your biochemical make-up, which takes place at the cellular level, where all bodily functions begin. I now believe that this test may be a significant step in the process to uncover underlying health problems when it comes to healing our body. This test can help you not only look at your CTS/RSI issue, but where your overall health trend is heading. Your health is everything, and you owe it to yourself to look for all the answers to your questions. You may be as surprised as she was and delighted by the outcome.

More About Hair Analysis

Hair analysis is an invaluable screening tool, which allows a correct program of nutritional support and supplementation to be designed for each individual's specific needs. Never before has there been available a "metabolic blueprint" with such a degree of applicable scientific accuracy.

Common Causes of a Mineral Imbalance are:

1. Improper diet
2. Taking vitamins and minerals that are not compatible with your current body chemistry
3. Medications
4. Birth control pills
5. STRESS
6. Accumulation of toxic metals from the environment, job or hobby
7. Inheritance of mineral patterns from parents

Conditions, which may result or be aggravated by a mineral imbalance, are:

1. Depression	11. Diabetes
2. Hypoglycemia	12. Musculo-Skeletal Disorders
3. Hyperactivity	13. Cardiovascular Disease
4. Headaches	14. Skin Rashes
5. Hypertension	15. Emotional Problems (PMS, Menopausal)
6. Arthritis	16. Allergies
7. Hair loss	17. Weight Issues
8. Thyroid Disturbance	18. Pregnancy Issues
9. Prostate Disorders	19. Hormonal Disturbances
10. Digestive Disturbance	20 Attention Deficit Disorder

Plus many more existing conditions… If you cannot find an explanation for your illness, or when the cause seems to be found but the therapy is not wholly effective, hair analysis can open up a new vista for the solving of your particular problem by recognizing your biochemical individuality.

To learn how you can order a Hair Analysis consult/test, refer to the Resource section of this book under Sports Touch.

*Information provided by Analytical Research Labs., Inc.

Kate's Recipe For Success

What do you think of when you think of growing older? You probably think of infirmity or disability – being tired or in pain or unable to do things. This feeling doesn't have to become a reality if you incorporate preventive therapies into your daily life. My recipe for preventing the aging process calls for this:

- Regular chiropractic care, once or twice a month, to ensure the stability of your skeletal structure

- Muscle therapy once a week or twice a month, to help maintain flexibility and mobility and to restore and maintain normal muscular functions. Muscle therapy is, in my opinion, the key component to keeping the body free of stress and pain. Therapeutic muscle therapy is not a luxury; it is a necessity!

- Acupuncture, once or twice a month, to help maintain your balance of vital energy and harmony throughout the body

- A balanced nutritional program, because the right fuel strengthens your immune system, and gives you energy

- Regular exercise, at least three times a week for thirty minutes at a time

- Meditation, to calm your mind and strengthen your spirit

- Plenty of rest, relaxation, and laughter!

The body is a magnificent machine. If you take care of it and don't wait to try to fix it until it is in pain and becomes sick, it will last a long time.

About The Author

Kate' Montgomery, is a Naturopathic Doctor (ND), H.H.P. (Holistic Health Practitioner), and a Certified Sports Massage Therapist. She is a Life and Wellness Consultant with a prior career as a respiratory therapist for twelve years. She has studied oriental medicine, natural herbal therapy, nutrition, and applied kinesiology. Kate' teaches practical and functional techniques that improve and revitalize the body, mind and spirit. Her clients include Olympic athletes, Ironman triathletes, and thousands who have suffered from carpal tunnel syndrome and other 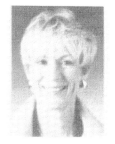 musculoskeletal disorders. Other books written by Kate' are Sports Touch: The Athletic Ritual, and Pain Free Back. Upcomming books include Hand Health, Artistic Ritual for Artists, and Hand Health for the Office and Industrial Athlete. She is a frequent guest on local, national, and international radio and television programs.

Resources

Information Sources

Informational Groups or Sites

Sports Touch

Web: http://www.sportstouch.com

Email: info@sportstouch.com

(866) 206-9066, ext. 8041

For more information on listings of RSD's resources, children and repetitive motion injuries, self-care for the back, strengthen the immune system, sports techniques for a better performance, and Sports Balm - herbal product to help heal the body, natural cancer treatment, the use of hair analysis in nutritional counseling, visit the Sports Touch.

Association of Repetitive Motion Syndromes (ARMS)

P.O. Box 471973

Aurora, Colorado 80047

Phone: 303-369-0803

Stephanie Barnes - Executive Director & Founder

Web site: www.CertifiedPST.com/arms

Email: Stephaniemara@hotmail.com

Newsletter, Advertising available, Association Sponsorship, and Donations, all highly appreciated. For a listing of support groups, please contact ARMS. Stephanie Barnes has dedicated her life to this disorder and to anyone who has ever suffered from carpal tunnel syndrome and other RSD's. Thank you for your support.

CTS Support Groups and Affiliate Associations

East Bay RSI Support Group

San Francisco, California

510-524-7127 (voice mail only)

The Repetitive Strain Injury Group of San Francisco

415-474-7060

Santa Clara Center for Occupational Safety and Health (SCCOSH)

Oversees two programs: Workers Acting Together for Change and Working Women's Leadership Project.

Concerned Advocates for the Rights of Employees (C.A.R.E.)

701-223-9207

Pennsylvania Injured Workers

http://members.aol.com/pfiw1

Pennsylvania Federation of Injured Workers (PFIW)

AMFMO153@access995.com

American Chronic Pain Association

www.acpa.org

Sorehand

www.ucsf.edu.sorehand

Listing of support groups from the newsletter: *Fibromyalgia & RSD's*

Chicago Area Committee on Occupational Safety and Health: SAFEWORKCHICAGO@AOL.COM

www.CACOSH.ORG

RSI Day Web Site

www.ctdrn.org/rsiday

CTD Resource Network, Inc.
www.ctdrn.org/

The Typing Injury Archive
www.tifaq.org

Harvard University RSI page
www.rsi.deas.harvard.edu/

Paul Marxhausen's RSI Page
www.engr.unl.edu/eeshop/rsi.html

Arthritis Foundation - Preventing CTS and Work Related Hand Pain
www.arthritis.org/resource/tips/preventCTS.shtml

RSI-ACTION (CNOT)
617-247-6827 (voice mail only)
Web site: www.rsiaction.org
Email: cnot@rsiaction.org
For information in the Boston area on RSI support groups, special events, speakers and more. All volunteer action group.

ADDITIONAL RESOURCES – THERAPY, HAND AND FINGER EXERCISERS

Upledger Institute
11211 Prosperity Farms Rd., Suite D-325
Palm Beach, FL 22410
Web: http://www.upledger.com
Email: upledger@upledger.com
Phone: 561-622-4334
Fax: 561-622-4771

Great Resource! Great Therapeutic Modality! Cranial Sacral Therapy is a gentle, hands-on method of evaluating and enhancing the functioning of a physiological body system called the craniosacral system. This therapy will help to improve the functioning of the central nervous system. Complements the body's natural healing process. This is great for anyone who is looking to find answers to why there body doing stuff they don't understand. It brings a new awareness to your healing. I love it.

Corporate Vision Consulting
Dr. Jeffrey Anshel
842 Arden Drive,
Encinitas, California 92024,
Phone: 619-944-1200,
Web: www.cvconsulting.com.
Email: eyedoc@adnc.com

For information about computer vision syndrome or other eye- or vision-related topics and to find an eye doctor in your area, this site can direct you.

Gookinaid HYDRALYTE
8525 –L Arjons Dr.
San Diego, CA 92126
Web: http://www.gookinaid.com
Email: info@gookinaid.com
Phone: 800-283-6505
Fax: 858-689-1859

Electrolyte replacement drink, is natural with no artificial sweeteners or additives. Search and Rescue teams call it the "Oral IV." Health professionals have recommended it for dehydration and illnesses, such as cold and flu, hypothermia, heat stress and more… It is the best! I have used it since 1985 to help my athletes recover from muscle soreness. To read more about this wonderful drink, go to their web site. Put in the code 7777 and mention this book.

Hand Health Unlimited

Finger Fitness™ Training Program

Greg Irwin – Creator

P.O. Box 13359

Hamilton, OH 45013

Web: http://www.handhealth.com

Email: info@handhealth.com

Phone: 888-868-42-63

Fax: 513-868-9038

Great Program and Resource! A program for strengthening the hands and fingers. Prevention and maintenance are the key and this is a good beginning. A regular program is a must to avoid repetitive strain injuries.

Healthy Referral Newspaper on-line

Marchia Carnicelli Minor and Thomas M. Katovsky-founders

Web: http://www.healthyreferral.com

Email: info@healthyreferral.com

Phone: 440-519-1889/779-7475

Fax: 440-519-1890

Great Resource! This nationally syndicated newspaper is full of resources for living a healthier life. Advertising what you do in this newspaper is a step toward saving the planet.

WisdomKing.com, Inc.

Web: http://www.wisdomking.com

Email: info@wisdomking.com

Digiflex Finger and Hand Exerciser (formerly the Grip Master) – Resistance comes in five levels: 1.5 lbs. (Yellow); 3.0 lbs. (Red); 5.0 lbs. (Green); 7.0 lbs. (Blue); 9.0 lbs. (Black).

I love this exerciser. Easy to use and it goes everywhere with me. I rate this as one of the best finger exercisers made. Every person who uses their fingers to hold a instrument or tool such as, a jeweler, dentist, dental hygienist, surgeon, musician, artist and more, should own this exerciser.

Great article written by APTA. You can read more on Hand and upper extremity conditions at this site.

http://www.apta.org/Consumer/ptandyourbody/hand/

Surgery is always a last resort and in most cases not necessary. The information in this article is worth reading. Good information for all who suffer with RSI.

NIOSH RECOMMENDATIONS

http://www.cdc.gov/niosh/ctsfs.html

Good Information by National Institute of Occupational Safety and Health (NIOSH). This reinforces what I say in my book. Additional NIOSH information about musculoskeletal disorders is available from the toll-free CDC Fax Information Service (1-888-232-3299); request fax document # 705005. NIOSH has also developed several publications that provide a description of NIOSH research on CTDs, including carpal tunnel syndrome, and practical ways to identify and evaluate musculoskeletal disorders. Copies of these publications, *Cumulative Trauma Disorders in the Workplace Bibliography* and *Elements of Ergonomics Programs*, are available free-of-charge from the NIOSH Publications Office while supplies last.

telephone **1-800-35-NIOSH** (1-800-356-4674)

fax 513-533-8573

www.cdc.gov/niosh/ctsfs.html

INFORMATION ON SOME EXTENSOR EXERCISOR DEVICES – WHERE TO FIND THEM

Flextend

www.repetitive-strain.com/treatment.html

Extensor muscle rehabilitation.

RGT Wrist Builder Lite -

http://www.paddleball.com/paddle/default.htm

Exercises designed to stretch and strengthen the flexor and extensor arm and hand muscles. Full range of movement.

OTHER EXERCISE DEVICES FOR THE FORARM AND HAND

www.tifaq.com/accessories/stretching.html

Information on several other devices marketed for muscle rehabilitation.

Specialty Therapy Equipment

George Kramer – President

8209 Ridder Ave.

Towson, MD 21204

gkramer@comcast.net

800-999-7839

An alternative device called a Neurometer, CPT/C, that measures nerve sensitivity and may catch problems before they develop into carpal tunnel syndrome. A noninvasive machine to screen for potential CTS problems. I used this myself and saw how quickly a reversal of nerve compression was using my program. We did a before and after and it verified for me that my program worked. A great addition to every companies health and safety program to help monitor their employees' recovery from RSI.

REFERENCE BOOKS:

How to Grow Fresh Air by Dr. B.C. Wolverton. Fifty House Plants that Purify your Home and Office.

Stop Your Pain Now by Dr. Walter H. Schmitt, D.C, D.I.B.A.K., D.A.B.C.N..

ISBN 0-97242280-0-3

Youth Inhancement System, Inc.

4770 Biscayne Blvd., Suite 1400

Miami, FL 33137

Web: www.stoppainusa.com

800-258-1930

Touch For Health by Dr. John Thie, .D.C.

ISBN 0-87516-180-4

The Myofascial Release Manual. by Carol J. Manheim.

Vision and Bodywork by Dr. Cleve Armstrong, O.D., M.P.H. 303-665-3200

ALTERNATIVE THERAPY COVERAGE

Some insurance companies are finally recognizing the benefits of alternative therapies. Sadly, in this age of technology, insurance companies do not recognize the fact that it would be more cost-effective to have you use these therapies on a regular basis than to have surgery – which is more expensive and often repeated later.

The insurance companies still do not understand how to use these therapies to allow you to maintain your health, well-being, and a continued productive and functional lifestyle. Most insurance companies would rather pay for you to have surgery – which unfortunately, for many people means ending up on the disability and semi-functional list for the rest of their lives.

To help make a change, write your Senators, Representatives and the Insurance Commissioner of your state, and demand change in the insurance laws. If you don't start asking for change, it will never happen. Citizens for Health, an advocate for change in the insurance system and for health care reform, can be found on the Internet. Contact them at www.citizens.org.

The following insurance companies offer a range of coverage for alternative therapies, such as chiropractic, massage, nutritional counseling, and others. Coverage varies form state to state, and individual policies vary as well. Check with your existing insurance carrier and employer to see if you have coverage for any of these therapies. If not, ask for consideration of expanded coverage.

For more information on how to get reimbursement for naturopathic services, contact the American Naturopathic Medical Association, at P.O. Box 96273, Las Vegas, Nevada, 89193, (702) 897-7053.

Aetna U.S. Health: acupressure, chiropractic, nutritional counseling; national coverage, (800) 872-3862.

Allina Health System: Medical Health Plan wellness programs: Acupressure, acupuncture, chiropractic; States - Minnesota, North Dakota, South Dakota, Wisconsin; (612) 992-2000.

Alternative Health Insurance Services: acupuncture, alternative birthing center/midwivery, ayurvedic medicine, bodywork/massage therapy, biofeedback, chiropractic, colon therapy, herbal medicine, homeopathy, nutrition counseling, naturopathy, oriental medicine, osteopathy, Transcendental Meditation; national coverage; (800) 966-8467.

America Medical Security, Health Care Choices plan: acupuncture, acupressure, biofeedback, chiropractor, Dean Ornish program, herbal medicine, hypnotherapy, homeopathy, (if practiced by M. D), massage, naturopathy, nutritional counseling; State-Arizona; (800) 232-5432.

American National: acupuncture, chiropractor, massage, nutritional counseling for diabetes; national coverage; (800) 899-6803.

American Western Life: wellness plans, acupuncture, acupressure, ayurvedic medicine, biofeedback, chiropractic, homeopathy, hypnotherapy, herbal medicine, naturopathy. States - Arizona, California, Colorado, New Mexico, Oregon, Utah; (800) 925-5323.

151

AmeriHealth: chiropractic, mental wellness program for drinking cessation; States - Connecticut, Delaware, Maine, New Hampshire, New Jersey, Pennsylvania, Texas; (800) 454-7651

Bienestar: acupuncture, chiropractic, nutritional counseling. State - New York; (888) 692-4363.

Blue Cross of California: acupressure, acupuncture, biofeedback, chiropractic, Dean Ornish program; State, California; (818) 703-2345

Blue Cross/Blue Shield of South Carolina: Dean Ornish program; State, South Carolina; (803) 788-0222

CHAMPUS: biofeedback; national coverage for military personnel; (800) 733-8387

CIGNA Health Care: acupuncture, biofeedback, chiropractic, nutritional counseling; national coverage; call the representative in your state.

Co-op America: chiropractic; national coverage; (800) 584-7336

CUNA Mutual Group: chiropractic, biofeedback, nutritional counseling, national coverage, including Puerto Rico; (800) 548-9390

Family Health Plan: chiropractic, nutritional counseling, physical therapy; States, Ohio, Michigan; (419) 241-6501

Fortis Benefits: acupressure, acupuncture, biofeedback, chiropractic, massage; most states; (800) 955-1586

Great West Assurance: acupressure, acupuncture, biofeedback, homeopathy, hypnotherapy, massage, naturopathy, nutritional counseling; national coverage; (800) 537-2033 ext. 4200

Guardian Life: naturopathy; national coverage; (800) 662-1006

Harvard Community Health Plan: offers discounts on personal health improvement program for stress-related illness, chronic disease, mood disorders; State, Massachusetts; (800) 543-7429

Harvard Pilgrim Health Care: chiropractic, nutritional counseling; States, Massachusetts, Rhode Island; (888) 333-4742

Health Partners Health Plan: acupuncture, guided imagery, herbal medicine (initial visit), homeopathy, nutritional counseling, osteopathy, craniosacral therapy, Therapeutic Touch, Trager/Feldenkrais therapies; Maricopa County, Arizona; (800) 351-1505

John Alden Life: acupuncture, chiropractic; national coverage; (800) 435-7969

Kaiser Permanente: acupressure, acupuncture, nutritional counseling, relaxation techniques, self-massage; national coverage; (800) 464-4000

Mutual of Omaha: acupuncture, Dean Ornish program, naturopathy; national coverage except Dean Ornish only in California, Iowa, Florida, Massachusetts, New York, South Carolina; (800) 456-0228

New England Mutual Life: acupressure, acupuncture, chiropractic; national coverage; (800) 237-4878

New York Life: acupuncture, herbal medicine, homeopathy, lifestyle counseling, nutritional counseling. States, New York, Connecticut; (800) 338-8113 and (718) 899-3600

Oxford Health Plans: acupuncture, chiropractic, massage, naturopathy, nutritional counseling, yoga; mail order catalog for herbal medicines; States, Connecticut, New Jersey, New York; (800) 444-6222

Pacific Mutual Life: naturopathy; national coverage; (800) 733-7020

Phoenix Home Life/Phoenix American Life:
acupuncture, biofeedback, chiropractic, nutritional
counseling; national coverage plus Puerto Rico,
Guam; (800) 343-0944

Physicians Health Services: naturopathy,
acupuncture; State, Connecticut; (800) 441-5741

Principal Mutual: acupressure, acupuncture,
biofeedback, chiropractic, Dean Ornish programs,
homeopathy, music and dance therapy (inpatient
only); national coverage; (800) 986-3343

Prudential: acupuncture, biofeedback, chiropractic,
massage, midwifery, naturopathy; national coverage;
(800) 346-3778

Sentry Life: acupressure, biofeedback, lifestyle
counseling; most states; (800) 533-7827

Suburban Health Plan: biofeedback, cardiac
reversal program (similar to Dean Ornish program),
chiropractic, homeopathy, naturopathy, holistic
psychotherapy, meditation/stress reduction, nutritional
counseling, yoga, acupressure, acupuncture, ayurvedic
medicine (M.D. only), bodywork, massage therapy;
State - Connecticut; (203) 734-4466

Trustmark: aromatherapy, chiropractic; Most states -
(800) 366-6663 or (800) 347-0889

Tufts Total Health Plan: nutritional counseling,
stress management; States - Massachusetts, Maine,
New Hampshire, Rhode Island; (800) 462-0224

Unicare: biofeedback chiropractic (only if
administered by M.D.), acupressure, acupuncture,
naturopathy; national coverage; (617) 572-7327

Woodmen Accident and Life: chemical dependency
counseling, chiropractic, counseling for mental
disorders; most states; (800) 869-0355

World: naturopathy; national coverage;
(800) 600-7760, ext. 3367

CARPAL TUNNEL SYNDROME ABSTRACTS FROM SCIENTIFIC RESEARCH FINDINGS

Ragberg, M: Morgenstern, H; Kelsh M.
Impact of occupations and job tasks on the prevalence of carpal tunnel syndrome.
National Institude of Occupational Health, Division of Work and Environmental Physiology, Solina, Sweden
Scand J Work Environmental Health 1992, Dec. 18 (6):337-45
Unique Identifier: Medline 93134348

Moore, JS
Carpal Tunnel Syndrome
Department of Preventive Medicine, Medical College of Wisconsin, Milwaukee, 53226
Occup. Med., 1992, Oct-Dec.; 7(4):741-63
Unique Identifier: Medline 93031140

Weiss, AP; Akelman, E.
Carpal Tunnel Syndrome: a review
Department of Orthopedics, Brown University, Providence, RI
RI Med.1992, June; 75(6):303-6
Unique Identifier: Medline 9236487

Chiu KY: Ng WF: Wong WB: Choi CH; Chow SP.
Acute carpal tunnel syndrome caused by pseudogout.
Department of Orthopedic Surgery, University of Hong Kong, Queen Mary Hospital.
J Hand Surg. (AM) 1992 Mar; 17(2):299-302
Unique Identifier: Medline 92226436

Skandalakis, JE; Colborn, GL; Skandalakis, PN; McCollam SM; Skandalakis, LJ.
The Carpal Tunnel Syndrome: Part II.
Centers for Surgical Anatomy & Technique, Emory University, Atlanta, GA 30322.
Am Surg. 1992 Feb;58(2):77-81
Unique Identifier: Medline 92197911

Szabo, RM; Madison M.
Carpal Tunnel Syndrome
Department of Orthopedics, University of California, Davis, Sacramento.
Orthop Clin. North Am 1992 Jan;23(1):103-9
Unique Identifier: Medline 92107436

Mascola, JR; Rickman, LS.
Infectious causes of carpal tunnel syndrome: cse report and review.
Infectious Diseases, Division, National Naval Medical Center, Bethesda, Maryland.
Rev. Infect. Dis. 1991 Sept-Oct: 13(5):911-7
Unique Identifier: Medline 92073810

Totten, PA; Hunter, JM.
Therapeutic techniques to enhance nerve gliding in thoracic outlet syndrome and carpal tunnel syndrome.
Hand Rehabilitation Center, Philadelphia, PA.
Hand Clin. 1991 Aug; 7(3):505-20
Unique Identifier: Medline 92042332

Baker, EL: Ehrenberg, RL.
Preventing the work-related carpal tunnel syndrome: Physician reporting and diagnostic criteria.
National Institute for Occupational Safety and Health, Centers for Disease Control, Atlanta, GA 30333
Ann. Intern. Med. 1990 Mar. 1;112(5):317-9
Unique Identifier: Medline 90165116

Hunter, JM
Recurrent carpal tunnel syndrome, epineural fibrous fixation, and traction neuropathy.
Jefferson Medical College, Thomas Jeffereson University, Philadelphia, PA.
Hand Clin. 1991 Aug: 7(3):491-504
Unique Identifier: Medline 92042331

Kuschner, SH; Ebramzadeh, E; Johnson, D: Brien, WW; Sherman, R.
Tinel's sign and Phalen's Test in carpal tunnel syndrome.
Department of Orthopedic Surgery, University of Southern California School of Medicine, Los Angeles, CA.
Orthopedics 1992 Nov:15(11):1297-302
Unique Identifier: Medline 93096704

Parmet,S; Lynm, C; Glass, M;
Carpal Tunnel Syndrome: a study comparing two treatments for carpal tunnel syndrome: the use of a wrist splint and carpal tunnel syndrome release surgery.
Jama, 2002:288:1310. September 11, 2002.

Glossary

ABDUCTOR DIGITI MINIMI: Muscle on the little finger side, palm side up, which is responsible for the movement of little finger.

ABDUCTOR POLLICIS BREVIS: Muscle on thumb side, palm side up. This muscle moves the thumb away from the palm. The neurolymphatic reflex point is under the left breast bone.

ADDUCTOR POLLICIS: Muscle on the thumb side, palm side up. This muscle contributes to the power of grasp or holding on to objects. The neurolymphatic reflex point is under the left breast bone.

ALVEOLI: Small chamber in the lungs, at the end of the bronchioles.

APPLIED KINESIOLOGY: Study of movement of muscles as applied to the evaluation of function.

ATROPHY: A wasting away due to nonuse, such as a wasting away (shrinking) of the muscles and bone that surround a joint, because of injury or disease.

BICEPS BRACHII: Front arm muscle. The neurolymphatic reflex point is in the space between fourth and fifth ribs, three inches from the breastbone.

BRACHIORADIALIS: Forearm muscle that flexes the elbow. The neurolymphatic reflex point is over the entire chest muscle.

BRONCHIOLES: Small channels or tubes branched off the bronchi, which are large passages conveying air to the lungs.

CARPAL LIGAMENT: A ligament that stretches across the transverse line of the wrist joint attaching to the carpal bones forming the carpal tunnel.

DIABETES: A general term referring to disorders characterized by inability to use or produce insulin, which is needed to process the sugar in food. A complication of diabetes is peripheral vascular disease.

DYNAMOMETER: An instrument that measures hand grip strength.

FLEXION: The movement of drawing two ends of a joint towards each other; the act of bending.

FLEXOR DIGITI MINIMI: Muscle on little finger, palm side up, which creates the flexion of the little finger. The neuro-lymphatic reflex point is under the left breastbone.

FLEXOR POLLICIS BREVIS: Muscle on the thumb, palm side up. This muscle helps create flexion of the thumb. The neuro-lymphatic reflex point is under the left breastbone.

HOOK OF HAMATE: Carpal or hand bone on the little finger side.

HYPEREXTENSION: Extreme bending backward, such as bending the wrist forward.

HYPERFLEXION: Extreme bending forward, such as bending the wrist backward.

LIGAMENT: A band of fibrous tissue that connects bones or cartilage, supporting and strengthening the joints.

LONTOPHORESIS: Involves electric current and stimulation.

MEDIAN NERVE: Located down the midline of the forearm, palm side up.

MISALIGNMENT: Not in a straight line, referring to the bony structure of the body.

MYOPATHY: Any disease of a muscle.

NERVE GANGLION: A group of nerve cell bodies forming a knot-like mass.

NEURAL: Related to nerves.

OPPONENS DIGITI MINIMI: Muscle on little finger side, palm side up, which rotates the little finger to meet the thumb. The neurolymphatic reflex point is under the left breastbone.

Ph: Measures acidity or alkalinity; scale ranges from 0 (acid) to 14 (alkaline). The pH of body fluids should be close to 7.4, or nearly neutral.

PHALEN' S TEST: A test to determine nerve entrapment by bending the wrist in extreme backward and forward movement.

PISIFORM BONE: A carpal or hand bone on the little finger side, closest to the wrist.

PRONATOR QUADRATUS: Wrist muscle that pronates the arm. The neurolymphatic reflex point is under the left breast.

PRONATOR TERES: Wrist muscle that pronates the arm and flexes the elbow. The neurolymphatic reflex point is under the left breast.

PROXIMAL: Close to any point of reference.

RADIUS BONE: A forearm bone located on the thumb side.

SUPINATOR: Arm muscle that rotates the arm inward. The neurolymphatic reflex point is located underneath the left breast.

TENDINITIS: Inflammation of a tendon.

TINEL'S TEST: A test to determine nerve entrapment (pinching or compression) by tapping the carpal ligament over the median nerve to elicit a pain response.

TRANSVERSE: Placed crosswise, at right angles, such as two bones at right angles to each other and a ligament stretched across them.

TRICEPS BRACHII: Arm muscle that extends forearm. The neurolymphatic reflex point is located in the seventh space between the ribs on the left, close to midline.

TRIGGER POINTS: A hypersensitive area in a muscle that is tender to the touch, and is brought on by physical and emotional stress.

When activated, a cycle of spasm and pain is set up in the musculature.

TUBERCLE OF TRAPEZIUM: A carpal or hand close to midline. bone, thumb side in front of the navicular tuberosity.

Glossary of Cumulative Trauma Disorders

BURSITIS - Inflammation of the bursae (small sacs of fluid in the body that help muscles and tendons glide over bone and ligaments).

CARPAL TUNNEL SYNDROME - Compression of the median nerve as it passes through the carpal tunnel.

CERVICAL RADICULOPATHY - Shoulder impairment caused by the partial dislocation of the spinal disks C4, C5, C6, and sometimes C7. Can be caused by post-traumatic neck and shoulder pain from a car accident or any trauma, such as from holding a phone to the ear with the shoulder.

CUBITAL TUNNEL SYNDROME - Entrapment of the ulnar nerve in the underarms. Can be caused by working excessively with bent elbow.

DEGENERATIVE DISC DISEASE - Chronic degeneration, narrowing, and hardening of a spinal disc, typically with cracking of the disc surface.

DEQUERVAIN'S DISEASE - Tendinitis of the thumb, typically affecting the base of the thumb. Causes pain when the thumb is moved or twisted.

DIGITAL NEURITIS - Inflammation of the nerves in the fingers caused by repeated contact or continuous pressure.

DIP JOINT: distal interphalangeal joint, the joint closest to the fingernail.

DISTAL ULNAR NEUROPATHY - Known as Guyon's canal or ulnar tunnel syndrome. Compression either at the wrist or elbow involving the ulnar nerve, which can cause numbness in the ring and little fingers. Very uncommon compared to carpal tunnel syndrome.

DOUBLE CRUSH SYNDROME – A double crush syndrome is a compression neuropathy of two areas, one usually distant from the other.

EPICONDYLITIS - Inflammation around an epicondyle, a bony part of the elbow. Forearm muscles are attached to the epicondyles by tendons, which can tear or become inflamed when overused. Called tennis elbow when on the outside of the elbow; golfers' elbow when on the inside of the elbow.

GANGLION CYST - Synovitis of the tendons of the flexors and extensors of the hand causing a bump under the skin. This is fluid buildup in the tendon, normally found at the wrist.

HERNIATED DISC - Rupturing or bulging of the spinal disc.

LIGAMENT SPRAIN - Tearing or stretching of a ligament (the fibrous connective tissue that helps support the bones) beyond its normal limits.

MECHANICAL BACK SYNDROME - Degeneration of the spinal facet joints

MUSCLE STRAIN - Overstretching or overuse of a muscle.

POSTURE STRAIN - Chronic stretching or overuse of neck muscles or related soft tissue.

PRONATOR SYNDROME - Compression of the median nerve where it passes between the two heads of pronator teres, which helps bend the elbow; sometimes involves the pronator quadratus muscle of the wrist.

RADIAL TUNNEL SYNDROME - Compression of the radial nerve in the forearm.

ROTATOR CUFF - A structure around the shoulder joint, including four tendons that connect to the fibrous capsule around the joint. The rotator cuff can be torn, or the surrounding tendons can be inflamed.

SULCAS ULNAR SYNDROME - Compression in the ulnar nerve caused by pressure on the ulnar bone. Can cause numbness, tingling, or contraction in the ring and little fingers.

SYNOVITIS - Inflammation of a tendon sheath.

TENDINITIS - Inflammation of a tendon.

TENOSYNOVITIS - Inflammation of the joint lining called the synovium.

TENSION NECK SYNDROME - Neck soreness, mostly related to static loading or tenseness of the neck muscles.

THORACIC OUTLET SYNDROME - Compression of nerves and blood vessels under the collarbone, brought about by misalignment of the thoracic vertebrae or specific cervical discs. Causes hand pain and can also cause pain and weakness in the shoulder or arm.

TRIGGER FINGER - Tendinitis of the finger, typically locking the tendon in its sheath and causing a snapping, jerking movement.

Index

Look to your Health; and if you have it, praise God, and value it next to a good
conscience, for health is the second blessing that we mortals are capable of;
a blessing that money cannot buy.

_____Izaak Walton

Self-Assessment

I recommended that you make multiple copies of the Self-Assessment Sheet for monitoring your progress.

Questionnaire

Do you think you have carpal tunnel syndrome? Yes____No____

Have you been diagnosed with carpal tunnel syndrome by a medical doctor?
Yes____No____

Have you ever had surgery for carpal tunnel syndrome?
Yes____No____

Have you ever had surgery for any other repetitive strain injury?
Yes____No____

Do you elicit any of these symptoms? Place an "X" next to those you are have now?

____pain in the neck?

____loss of sense of touch in the hands and/or fingers?

____tingling or numbness in hands and/or fingers?

____pain in the shoulders at night after sleep?

____loss of grip strength in one or both hands?

____pain in the wrist joint when bending the wrist?

____swelling in the wrist?

____nodules or "ganglion cyst" at the wrist?

____pain in the elbow?

____can't unscrew a jar lid?

____dropping objects a lot?

____difficult to brush your hair or button a blouse?

SELF-ASSESSMENT TESTS

RATE YOUR OVERALL CONDITION

   Before you begin, rate your overall condition of your arms and hands. 0 – 10, where "0" is NO problems and "10" is severe problems. (Circle one)

Right Hand

0 1 2 3 4 5 6 7 8 9 10

Left Hand

0 1 2 3 4 5 6 7 8 9 10

TEST 1. TINEL'S TEST

BEFORE CORRECTIONS

After tapping my finger over the carpal tunnel area, I felt
(Place an X next to your current symptoms)

Right Hand
____pain   ____slight pain   ____moderate pain
____strong pain   ____severe pain

Left Hand
____pain   ____slight pain   ____moderate pain
____strong pain   ____severe pain

AFTER CORRECTIONS

Right Hand
____pain   ____slight pain   ____moderate pain
____strong pain   ____severe pain

Left Hand
____pain   ____slight pain   ____moderate pain
____strong pain   ____severe pain

TEST 2. PHALEN'S TEST

BEFORE CORRECTIONS

After bending my wrists both ways (extreme hyper-extension and hyper-flexion of the wrists, I felt:

(Place an "X" next to your current symptoms)

Right Hand
____pain   ____slight pain   ____moderate pain
____strong pain   ____severe pain

Left Hand
____pain   ____slight pain   ____moderate pain
____strong pain   ____severe pain

AFTER CORRECTIONS

(Place an "X" next to your current symptoms)

Right Hand
____pain   ____slight pain   ____moderate pain
____strong pain   ____severe pain

Left Hand
____pain   ____slight pain   ____moderate pain
____strong pain   ____severe pain

TEST 3. MUSCLE MONITORING

With a partner, assess your hand strength. Follow the Directions in Chapter 2 on how to do the Muscle Monitoring Tests.

BEFORE CORRECTIONS

Right Hand Palm-up:
_____a) The thumb and little finger came apart a very small amount (you could see a little space between them)
_____b) The Thumb and little finger came apart more than a 1/4 inch or more.
_____c) The thumb and little finger did not come apart at all.

Right Hand Palm-down:
_____a) The thumb and little finger came apart a very small amount (you could see a little space between them)
_____b) The Thumb and little finger came apart more than a 1/4 inch or more.
_____c) The thumb and little finger did not come apart at all.

Left Hand Palm-up
_____a) The thumb and little finger came apart a very small amount (you could see a little space between them)
_____b) The Thumb and little finger came apart more than a 1/4 inch or more.
_____c) The thumb and little finger did not come apart at all.

Left Hand Palm-down:
_____a) The thumb and little finger came apart a very small amount (you could see a little space between them)
_____b) The Thumb and little finger came apart more than a 1/4 inch or more.
_____c) The thumb and little finger did not come apart at all.

AFTER CORRECTIONS

Right Hand Palm-up:
_____a) The thumb and little finger came apart a very small amount (you could see a little space between them)
_____b) The Thumb and little finger came apart more than a 1/4 inch or more.
_____c) The thumb and little finger did not come apart at all.

Right Hand Palm-down:
_____a) The thumb and little finger came apart a very small amount (you could see a little space between them)
_____b) The Thumb and little finger came apart more than a 1/4 inch or more.
_____c) The thumb and little finger did not come apart at all.

Left Hand Palm-up
_____a) The thumb and little finger came apart a very small amount (you could see a little space between them)
_____b) The Thumb and little finger came apart more than a 1/4 inch or more.
_____c) The thumb and little finger did not come apart at all.

Left Hand Palm-down:
_____a) The thumb and little finger came apart a very small amount (you could see a little space between them)
_____b) The Thumb and little finger came apart more than a 1/4 inch or more.
_____c).The thumb and little finger did not come apart at all.

TEST 4. FINGER PAD SENSITIVITY – SENSORY PERCEPTION

I rate my sensitivity: 0 – 10, where "0" is NO feeling and "10" is the most sensitive (Circle one)

BEFORE CORRECTIONS
Right Hand

0 1 2 3 4 5 6 7 8 9 10

Left Hand

0 1 2 3 4 5 6 7 8 9 10

AFTER CORRECTIONS

I rate my sensitivity: 0 – 10, where "0" is NO feeling and "10" is the most sensitive (Circle one)

Right Hand

0 1 2 3 4 5 6 7 8 9 10

Left Hand

0 1 2 3 4 5 6 7 8 9 10

TEST 5. PERCEIVED GRIP STRENGTH

BEFORE TEST
When I squeeze my fist firmly together, I rate my Perceived Grip Strength on a scale from 0 – 10, with "0" indicating NO strength and "10" indicating the strongest my hands feel at this time. (Circle one)

0 1 2 3 4 5 6 7 8 9 10

AFTER CORRECTIONS
When I squeeze my fist firmly together, I rate my Perceived Grip Strength on a scale from 0 – 10, with "0" indicating NO strength and "10" indicating the strongest my hands feel at this time. (Circle one)

0 1 2 3 4 5 6 7 8 9 10

TEST 6. MUSCLE PALPATION

BEFORE MUSCLE THERAPY

Rate your perception of your muscle tightness as you palpate your hand and forearm muscles. 0 – 10, where "0" is very relaxed and "10" is extremely tight and ropey. (Circle one)

Right Hand/Forearm
0 1 2 3 4 5 6 7 8 9 10

Left Hand/Forearm
0 1 2 3 4 5 6 7 8 9 10

AFTER MUSCLE THERAPY

Right Hand/Forearm

0 1 2 3 4 5 6 7 8 9 10

Left Hand/Forearm

0 1 2 3 4 5 6 7 8 9 10

TEST 7. PAIN LEVEL

BEFORE MUSCLE THERAPY – PAIN LEVEL
Rate the pain level in your muscles, where"0" is no pain and "10" is extreme pain. (Circle one)

Right Hand/Forearm

0 1 2 3 4 5 6 7 8 9 10

Left Hand/Forearm

1 1 2 3 4 5 6 7 8 9 10

AFTER MUSCLE THERAPY – PAIN LEVEL

Right Hand/Forearm

1 1 2 3 4 5 6 7 8 9 10

Left Hand/Forearm

1 2 3 4 5 6 7 8 9 10

RATE YOUR OVERALL CONDITION

After you have done all the self assessment tests and 12 Step Corrections, rate your overall condition of your arms and hands. 0 – 10, where "0" is NO improvement and "10" is no pain and no muscle tightness. (Circle one)

First day
Right Hand/Forearm
0 1 2 3 4 5 6 7 8 9 10

Left Hand/Forearm
0 1 2 3 4 5 6 7 8 9 10

Second Day
Right Hand/Forearm
0 1 2 3 4 5 6 7 8 9 10

Left Hand/Forearm
0 1 2 3 4 5 6 7 8 9 10

One Week
Right Hand/Forearm
0 1 2 3 4 5 6 7 8 9 10

Left Hand/Forearm
0 1 2 3 4 5 6 7 8 9 10

One Month
Right Hand/Forearm
0 1 2 3 4 5 6 7 8 9 10

Left Hand/Forearm
0 1 2 3 4 5 6 7 8 9 10

I recommend that you keep a journal of your progress. This will help to remind you that you are making strides toward healing your body. You have my permission to make copies of this sheet. Good Luck and Many Blessings for Your Recovery!

Please send copies of your self-assessment to Sports Touch. This is on-going research for me. Please email only to info@sportstouch.com. Thank you. Kate'

I want to especially thank Jim Schmidt, director of the Bellevue Massage School in Bellevue, WA for his help in writing this questionnaire and self-assessment sheet and for his on-going research using my program. He proved over and over again that a non-invasive approach and The Montgomery Method worked in reducing symptoms of CTS/RSI in over 80% of the people he worked with in various companies in his area.

REEDSBURG PUBLIC LIBRARY
370 Vine Street
Reedsburg, WI 53959